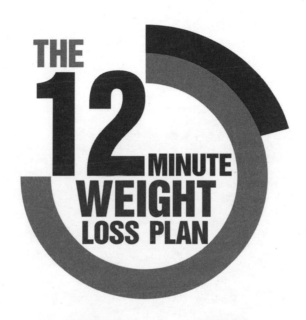

THE 12 MINUTE WEIGHT LOSS PLAN

DR MICHAEL SPIRA

piatkus

PIATKUS

First published in Great Britain in 2015 by Piatkus

Copyright © Dr Michael Spira 2015

The moral right of the author has been asserted.

A CIP catalogue record for this book
is available from the British Library.

ISBN 978-0-349-40539-1

Illustrations by D.R. ink

Typeset in Albertina by M Rules
Printed and bound in Great Britain by
Clays Ltd, St Ives plc

Papers used by Piatkus are from well-managed forests
and other responsible sources.

MIX
Paper from
responsible sources
FSC® C104740

Piatkus
An imprint of
Little, Brown Book Group
100 Victoria Embankment
London EC4Y 0DY

An Hachette UK Company
www.hachette.co.uk

www.piatkus.co.uk

ABOUT THE AUTHOR

Dr Michael Spira (MB, BS, MRCS, LRCP) qualified as a doctor at St Bartholomew's Hospital. After initially specialising in eye surgery, he became a GP and eventually the senior partner in a large family practice.

After his weight crept up to over 1 stone (6.3kg) overweight, he tried unsuccessfully to lose weight by following various diets until he worked out an approach that *did* work. This approach was published by Penguin as *How to Lose Weight Without Really Dieting*. Dr Spira has subsequently written other diet books. He has also been an adviser to the UK government on an obesity programme, a member of the Association of the Study of Obesity and the National Obesity Forum and a medical consultant on diet and lifestyle at a leading group of wellness clinics.

Besides his many books and articles, Dr Spira has regularly featured as a guest on national TV and radio, including as a medical expert on BBC1's *Kilroy*, ITV's *GMT* and *The Gloria Hunniford Show*.

To all those who struggle with their weight

DISCLAIMER

Exercise is not without its risks and may result in injury. Before attempting a new exercise consider your overall health, strength and flexibility in order to decide if a particular exercise is suitable for you. Remember, almost any exercise can result in personal injury. To reduce the risk of injury, it is advisable to consult your doctor before beginning an exercise programme. Any advice given in this book is not a substitute for medical consultation. As with any exercise programme, if at any point during your workout you begin to feel faint, dizzy, or have physical discomfort, you should stop immediately and consult a physician.

CONTENTS

ACKNOWLEDGEMENTS

THANK YOU to the following individuals, without whose contributions and support this book would not have been published: my agent, Jane Graham Maw, of Graham Maw Christie; Anne Lawrance at Piatkus, who championed this book; and Jan Cutler, who is probably the best copy editor a writer could wish for and who made many suggestions and corrected many mistakes. All the errors that remain are my sole responsibility.

WHO IS THIS BOOK FOR?

ANSWER YES OR NO to the following questions:

▶ Are you overweight? And do you want to lose weight?

▶ Do you enjoy your food? But hate the idea of going on a diet?

▶ Do you find exercise boring? Or do you find it difficult to find the time to do it? And are you physically lazy?

If you answered yes to all three questions, this book is definitely for you. Even if you didn't answer yes to all three – or indeed any – of the questions, this book is probably also for you. That's because in this day and age many of us have grown to love and appreciate our food while at the same time our busy lives make it difficult to spend hours each week in the gym or pummelling roads to keep trim.

At the time of writing, this book is unique. It is the only book that provides a unique and proven guide to weight loss without the need to go on a special diet or to spend hours exercising. All you have to do is to cut a few corners rather than having to do anything really drastic. At the same time the programme gives you a road to good health and fitness.

It is based on validated research and the sources of much of that research are given in the book.

INTRODUCTION

WHY, YOU MIGHT ASK, do we need yet another book on how to lose weight? The simple answer is that so far no one has got the answer completely right. So what's been going wrong until now? To answer that we need to look at two issues: diet and exercise. We all know that to lose weight you have to combine these two, but there's a right and a wrong way for each. Or, perhaps more accurately, there's a more effective way and a less effective way for each.

The myth with diet is that all you have to do is to cut calories or cut fat (unless you're an Atkins fan, in which case you increase your fat!). But, as this book will show you, this is not an effective dietary approach for weight loss. Yes, of course, you have to cut calories in some way, but it's *how* you do it that is crucial. Compared to the large amounts of carbs that people generally eat today, this book will show you how to lower carbs gently, allowing you to follow a diet that is closer to the one that was eaten by most people 40 or 50 years ago when obesity was rare and people were much healthier.

The myth with exercise is that to lose weight you have to put in lots of hours, preferably at a gym or jogging outside in all weathers, or swimming the equivalent of the English Channel every week. Again, this is just not true.

I presume the reason you're looking at this book is because of that phrase '12-minute' in the title – it's the most attractive part for most people, so I won't go into the dietary approach here, as there's lots about that later in the book. For now, I think it's sufficient to say that the diet is simple and delicious and won't leave you hungry. Let's focus for a moment on the 12-minutes-of-exercise part. What's that all about?

The buzzword is HIIT – that stands for high-intensity interval training. Instead of spending hours each week running around a park or on a treadmill, you spend a few minutes doing *really intensive* exercise, and you do this three times a week.

What do I mean by intense though? Imagine running for a bus. It's vital you catch it. Perhaps it's the last bus home. You run as fast as you can for 30 seconds or so and catch it before the doors close. You flash your ticket or card at the driver and then spend the next 30 seconds panting your way to recovery. Then you do the same again – 30 seconds fast and furious followed by 30 seconds relaxing. You go through this cycle four times – that's four minutes. Do this three times a week and there's your 12 minutes of high-intensity interval training.

Why does this fantastic time-saving way of exercise work? The answer is, we don't fully know. Sports physiologists are working to find the answers as I write this. HIIT has been around for a while, mostly used by athletes, but it's only in the last few years that its value for everybody has been recognised. The HIIT sessions in this book bring the technique bang up to date and will appeal to anyone who wants to get fit and healthy, regardless of their age.

At least part of the reason why we become fat – and certainly a lot of the reason why we can't shift that fat – is to do with inflammation in our body, especially a part of our brain called the hypothalamus. Why it becomes inflamed is another story, but it has a lot to do with the kind of food we eat. The key is that if we can reduce the inflammation we can increase the sensitivity of the hypothalamus to a hormone called leptin. This is made by fat tissue and acts on the brain to regulate our food intake and body weight. The more sensitive our brain is to leptin, the easier it is to lose and control weight. And it seems that exercise, especially HIIT, reduces inflammation and improves leptin sensitivity.

That's not the whole story, however. Another important factor in weight control is the burning of sugar in our bodies. Sugar is stored as glycogen in our muscles. Conventional exercise, such as jogging, uses around 40 per cent of the muscles in our body. HIIT, on the other hand, can use as much as *80 per cent* of our body's muscles. This means that HIIT can result in twice as much sugar being burned off.

A great bonus of HIIT is that its fat-burning effectiveness continues long after you've finished the exercise. That's why I recommend HIIT three times a week on alternate days rather than every day. Another bonus for this kind of exercise is that HIIT is a great way to improve your fitness.

Later in this book we'll look at some of the research that supports the effectiveness of HIIT, and of course we'll look at some of the different ways we can use it.

HOW I FOUND THE IDEAL WEIGHT-CONTROL METHOD

Before we start on the programme itself, here's a little about me. I qualified as a doctor at St Bartholomew's Hospital in London, one of the world's oldest and most established medical teaching hospitals. After initially specialising in eye surgery, I decided I was far more interested in treating the whole person, not just their eyes, so I decided to go into general practice and eventually became the senior partner in a large family practice.

One day I realised that my weight had crept up and I had become 1 stone (6.3kg) overweight. I tried to lose weight by following the popular diets of the day, which were crude calorie-controlled diets – this was the 1970s – but nothing seemed to work. Eventually, I worked out an approach that did work, and I wrote it down as a book. The publisher, Penguin, loved the book and it sold well both in the UK and the US.

Over the years I have held the following roles:

▶ A medical consultant to some of the UK's leading groups of slimming clubs and magazines.

▶ An adviser to the UK government on an obesity programme.

▶ An adviser to a Scottish working party on obesity.

▶ A member of the Association of the Study of Obesity.

▶ A member of the National Obesity Forum.

▶ A medical consultant at a leading group of wellness clinics where advice on lifestyle and diet were key issues.

▶ The author of many books and articles on nutrition and obesity.

▶ A frequent guest on national TV and radio to discuss obesity.

You can find more information in my Wikipedia entry at: en.wkipedia.org/wiki/Michael_Spira.

Over the years I've seen hundreds of diets and slimming books come and go, but how many of them have been successful in the long term? Quite simply, very few, mostly because it's not so much the diet as what happens afterwards once you've reached your target weight.

In recent years more and more of my patients have come across the very first book I wrote in the 1970s. They've told me that they've followed the principles and, guess what? The method still works! Countless patients have asked me why the book is out of print, and this is finally what prompted me to look again at the book and update it to bring it firmly into the 21st century and to benefit from all the latest research into overweight and obesity. I was also especially interested in the latest research into the effects of exercise on body weight.

As I hope you'll find, the message of this book is simple: it isn't necessary to 'go on a diet' in order to lose weight. In fact, it's positively counter-productive to do so. Nor is it necessary to spend hours in a gym working out. The key to successful and permanent weight loss is a combination of lifestyle, properly focused very-short-duration exercise, and a few very small, subtle changes to your diet.

My first slimming book, which became a bestseller, was called *How to Lose Weight Without Really Dieting*. Over the years I have had many patients who have successfully lost weight and kept that weight. My methods, described in that book and my subsequent ones, are truly tried and tested, easy to follow and can easily be fitted into a busy lifestyle. This book – *The 12-Minute Weight-Loss Plan* – carries on from where that first one left off.

I truly believe that this book provides for most people the most effective way to lose weight, and to keep that weight off, without going on a restrictive diet or spending hours working out in a gym. In my experience the method described herein, if applied and followed, is likely to be successful for at least 80 per cent of people.

Wishing you good luck and good health,

Michael Spira

Part One

WHY ARE WE OVERWEIGHT?

Chapter One

GETTING YOUR FACTS STRAIGHT AND LOOKING FORWARD TO CHANGE

I F YOU ARE ONE OF the many people today who are struggling to keep their weight under control, this chapter will help you to get on the road to making real changes that will benefit you in many ways. When you follow the programme I describe in this book, you will lose weight and feel great.

LET'S FACE FACTS

It's headline news these days that we're all getting fatter, but most people are searching for a way to solve this problem. Let's start with the facts. Here's the bad news:

FACT Obesity is one of the biggest health threats to the UK population.

FACT The UK is top of the European league table for obesity in women.

FACT The UK holds second place in the European league table for obesity in men.

FACT The UK has more obese young people than any European country.

FACT Three-fifths of adults in England are either overweight or obese.

FACT Almost a quarter of four- to five-year-olds are overweight or obese.

FACT Most people are heavier than they would have been 20 years ago – even thin people.

FACT If present trends continue, three-fifths of all men, half of all women, and a quarter of all children will be obese by 2050.

And now for some good news:

FACT A weight loss of just 10 per cent leads to enormous health benefits.

And the most startling fact of all:

FACT *Overweight and obesity are lifelong conditions* – just like diabetes and high blood pressure.

You can't cure obesity, but you can control it. Unless you control it with a good long-term eating programme combined with lifestyle changes, regardless of how much weight you have lost, it will return.

The American Academy of Nutrition and Dietetics (the world's largest organisation of food and nutrition professionals) says that 'successful weight management to improve overall health for adults requires a lifelong commitment to healthful lifestyle behaviours emphasizing sustainable and enjoyable eating practices and daily physical activity.'

This is where this book comes in.

WHAT MAKES A GOOD WEIGHT-LOSS PROGRAMME?

Which would you rather follow in order to lose weight? A trendy diet with expensive diet foods? A diet that's all about denial and restriction? A diet that requires you to spend hours in the gym each week? Or a diet that allows you to eat a wide range of foods, including some of your favourites, and still lose weight? A diet that is easy, painless, realistic and suited to you as an individual and your lifestyle? A diet that requires only a small amount of time doing exercise?

The best weight-loss programme is the one that suits us the best, the one that takes into account our likes and dislikes – and how much time we have to prepare our food and to take exercise.

Let's face it, though, it's easy to lose weight in the short term: just cut the calories and most of our favourite foods, and we'll get there. But can we stick to that? And would we want to? The answer is, of course not.

So what is a good weight-loss plan, and what are its features? Let's think about seven key essentials:

1. It must work: we must lose weight!

2. It must be sustainable. An eating plan is like a pet dog – it's for life.

3. It must include the foods we enjoy.

4. It mustn't ban any food – with one or two possible minor exceptions.

5. It must be nutritionally balanced. A healthy diet can boost energy, keep our immune system strong, and improve our skin, hair and nails.

6. It must be easy for us to manage in our lifestyle – most of us don't want to have to cook a complicated dish after a long day at work. And most of us shudder at the thought of having to take lots of exercise.

7. It must be flexible – birthdays, Christmas and Passover happen!

First we need to understand why we put on excess weight to start with and to recognise what happens in our bodies when we eat certain foods. That way we can better appreciate how to move forward towards losing weight and keeping trim.

Chapter Two

WHAT IS OVERWEIGHT – AND DOES IT MATTER?

WHAT DO WE MEAN when we say we are fat? What does it mean to be overweight or obese? It means having more body fat than is generally reckoned to be healthy for us. Contrary to what you might read in magazines, there is no single ideal weight for each height. Instead, there is a range of healthy weights based on a measurement called the body mass index (BMI). This is calculated by dividing your weight in kilograms (without clothes) by the square of your height in metres (without shoes). It sounds complicated, but it is really quite simple.

For someone 1.7m (5ft 7in) tall who weighs 70kg, their BMI is:

$$70 \div 1.7 \times 1.7 = 24$$

The World Health Organization has devised a simple scale:

BMI 18.5–25.0 = normal weight

BMI 25.1–30.0 = overweight

BMI 30.1–40.0 = obese

BMI 40.1 or more = morbidly obese

If maths isn't your favourite subject, don't worry. I've done the calculation for you below. For both men and women, healthy BMIs are between 20 and 25, and the tables below are based on this range. Weights above and below this range are unhealthy. For someone whose weight is at the upper end of the range there is no medical need to lose further weight. As to looking good in your favourite bikini – that's another matter!

BMI RANGES IN IMPERIAL MEASUREMENTS

Height	From	To
4ft 8in	6st 6lb (90lb)	8st 0lb (112lb)
4ft 9in	6st 9lb (93lb)	8st 4lb (116lb)
4ft 10in	6st 12lb (96lb)	8st 8lb (120lb)
4ft 11in	7st 1lb (99lb)	8st 12lb (124lb)
5ft 0in	7st 5lb (103lb)	9st 3lb (129lb)
5ft 1in	7st 8lb (106lb)	9st 7lb (133lb)
5ft 2in	7st 12lb (110lb)	9st 11lb (137lb)
5ft 3in	8st 1lb (113lb)	10st 1lb (141lb)
5ft 4in	8st 4lb (116lb)	10st 5lb (145lb)
5ft 5in	8st 8lb (120lb)	10st 10lb (150lb)
5ft 6in	8st 12lb (124lb)	11st 1lb (155lb)
5ft 7in	9st 2lb (128lb)	11st 6lb (160lb)

▶

Height	From	To
5ft 8in	9st 6lb (132lb)	11st 11lb (165lb)
5ft 9in	9st 10lb (136lb)	12st 2lb (170lb)
5ft 10in	10st 0lb (140lb)	12st 7lb (175lb)
5ft 11in	10st 4lb (144lb)	12st 12lb (180lb)
6ft 0in	10st 8lb (148lb)	13st 3lb (185lb)
6ft 1in	10st 12lb (152lb)	13st 8lb (190lb)
6ft 2in	11st 2lb (156lb)	14st 0lb (196lb)
6ft 3in	11st 6lb (160lb)	14st 5lb (201lb)

BMI RANGES IN METRIC MEASUREMENTS

Height	From	To
1.40m	39kg	49kg
1.42m	40kg	50kg
1.44m	42kg	52kg
1.46m	43kg	53kg
1.48m	44kg	55kg
1.50m	45kg	56kg
1.52m	46kg	58kg
1.54m	48kg	60kg
1.56m	49kg	61kg
1.58m	50kg	63kg
1.60m	51kg	64kg
1.62m	52kg	66kg
1.64m	54kg	67kg
1.66m	55kg	69kg

▶

Height	From	To
1.68m	56kg	71kg
1.70m	58kg	73kg
1.72m	59kg	74kg
1.74m	61kg	76kg
1.76m	62kg	78kg
1.78m	63kg	80kg
1.80m	65kg	82kg
1.82m	66kg	83kg
1.84m	68kg	85kg
1.86m	69kg	86kg
1.88m	71kg	88kg
1.90m	72kg	90kg

DOES BEING OVERWEIGHT REALLY MATTER?

Apart from a small minority of obese people who are in self-denial, most people would agree that being overweight or obese is bad for your health and, for most people, it is also bad for their self-esteem. Apart from the health consequences, it is an inescapable fact that employment prospects can be affected if you are seriously overweight. Overweight people are assumed by many to be greedy, lazy or habitually eating unhealthy food, although that's not necessarily the case. They are often criticised by the government and media as well as others on internet forums, and this can be very distressing.

Among the health consequences of overweight and obesity the following are the most common:

► Heart disease

► Stroke

► Type-2 diabetes

► Musculoskeletal disorders, especially osteoarthritis (often termed 'wear and tear' degeneration of the joints)

► Some cancers (colon, breast, the lining of the womb)

Childhood obesity is very much on the increase and, for the first time, doctors are now seeing children with type-2 diabetes as a direct consequence of obesity. Other health issues include breathing difficulties, high blood pressure, disability in adulthood and premature death.

WHY IT'S IMPORTANT TO KNOW YOUR WAIST MEASUREMENT

Being overweight is a risk to our health. The height–weight tables above give you a fairly good idea of whether you are under-weight, normal weight, overweight or obese, but they're not an infallible guide. Healthy athletes in training often have a high muscle mass, which results in their BMI often being higher than would be considered normal – but that's not unhealthy.

If we are carrying excess body *fat*, however, as well as knowing how much there is, it is important to know where in our body that fat is located. In particular, fat around our waist carries the greatest risk for health.

You can find out if you are carrying excess fat in your abdomen simply by measuring your waist. To do this, first stand up, then find the point which is halfway between the top of your hip bone and the bottom of your rib cage, vertically below your armpit. (Incidentally, this is not necessarily where your umbilicus, or belly-button, is.) Now look at the following figures:

	Increased health risk	Substantial health risk
Men	94cm (37in) or more	102cm (40in) or more
Women	80cm (32in) or more	88cm (35in) or more

If your waist is greater than the levels above, it is even more important to lose weight. The good news is that the eating approach in this book is particularly good at helping to get rid of a large tummy – as well as shedding the bits you don't want on your hips and thighs.

HOW OFTEN SHOULD WE WEIGH OURSELVES?

Most doctors and dieticians will tell you to weigh yourself once a week. Let me tell you why I think that's completely wrong.

I don't believe there is one answer that suits everyone and every situation. For a start, it depends on how much weight you need to lose. And it also depends on whether you're still losing weight or just maintaining weight loss. I'll explain.

If you are very overweight, you will lose weight more quickly than someone with only a few pounds to lose. Also, you probably need a lot of motivation and feedback. Why wait a whole week when the likelihood is that you're going to see measurable results every two to three days? When you get closer to your target weight, however, you'll find that your weight comes off more slowly. At that point weighing yourself once a week makes good sense.

Now let's look at the situation where you've lost your weight and you just want to make sure you don't pile it back on again. Is it easier to lose the 1 pound (450g) or 2 pounds (900g) that you've accidentally gained? Is it easier to lose 2 pounds (900g) or 4 pounds (1.8kg)? Well, the only way to spot that 1 pound (450g) before it's crept up to become 2 pounds (900g) or that 2 pounds before it's reached 4 pounds (1.8kg) is to weigh yourself every day. Small corrections are much easier to make than large ones.

A final tip: always weigh yourself at the same time of day. The best time is as soon as you get out of bed, after you've been to the toilet and before you've had breakfast.

Gaining weight is not always as simple and straightforward as just eating too much or not exercising enough, as I will explain in the next chapter.

Chapter Three

WHAT MAKES US BECOME FAT?

THERE IS NO SINGLE REASON WHY we gain weight. The body is complex and affected by hormones, our genes and our environment. Understanding the influences will help us find ways to overcome the problem of weight gain and to kick-start the process of weight loss.

THE LEPTIN STORY

What makes us become overweight or obese? Until a few years ago, doctors believed that our body's fat stores depended on the balance between:

1. Our intake of energy; that is, how many calories we ate

   and

2. Our energy output; that is, how many calories we burned off through physical activity and our metabolism.

But recent research has shown that this is not true. There is a third factor, which is very important:

3. How *efficiently* we burn off calories.

In other words, we now know that there are not two but *three* energy-balance components. We also now know that these three components are controlled by underlying *genetic* and *physiological* mechanisms.

In the early 1900s there was a major breakthrough: the discovery of the hormone leptin. We'll look at this more closely later in this chapter. But for now, the main point is that, along with other mechanisms, leptin protects us against starvation. It works hard to maintain our body-fat stores. In evolutionary terms, it helps to set us up for hibernation. The result is that it 'messes up' the traditional 'calories in versus calories out' equation.

Why does leptin seem to work so efficiently in some of us and therefore keep us fat while in others it works inefficiently with the result that those people are thin? We'll look at why in the next two chapters.

NATURE OR NURTURE?

We all know people who seem only to have to look at a doughnut to pile on the weight and others who apparently stuff their faces until the cows come home and never put on an ounce. How infuriating is that? What is the reason this happens? The chorus always goes up: 'It's all in the genes!', but is it?

To answer that question, the *British Medical Journal* (*BMJ*) published a head-to-head debate in 2012: are the causes of obesity primarily environmental?

The nurture argument (or, it isn't our genes, it's our environment)

A resounding yes was given by Dr John Wilding, professor of medicine and obesity specialist at Liverpool University. He says that while genetics undoubtedly play a role, gene defects are either rare or have only a very small effect, accounting for at most 6½ pounds (3kg) greater weight. The increase in obesity has mainly occurred over the past 30 years and has been seen in most parts of the world. Such a rapid change cannot be due to genetic changes, but the evidence that the environment has changed is overwhelming. You only have to look at the substantial shifts in the production and availability of food, occurring at the same time as changes in our physical environment that encourage a sedentary lifestyle. The relative cost of energy-dense foods high in fat, salt, sugar and refined carbs has fallen while the cost of healthier options has increased. This is partly why obesity is more common in those on lower incomes. The food industry, now an unhealthy alliance of producers and marketeers, has successfully promoted energy-dense foods. The healthy-eating advice from the 1970s also encouraged us all to fill up on carbohydrates, so even people who are eating a healthy diet can put on weight because they are eating more carbs than they would have done in the 1950s and 1960s.

All the while, physical activity has declined, and time spent being sedentary has increased. This is largely due to changes in transport, especially the increased use of the car, and in time spent being inactive during work and leisure time; for example, the increased time spent watching television, using computers or playing computer games, and so on.

Professor Wilding summarised it as follows: 'Obesity is a complex disorder with both genetic and environmental causes. The predominant driver is environmental.'

Professor Wilding could have pointed to another interesting observation: plastic food packaging and its role in encouraging obesity. A few years ago, the University of Sheffield held a workshop, 'Obesity Unwrapped: plastic food packaging and obesity', which was organised by Clare Renton, research fellow in public health and author of a 2012 *BMJ* article, 'Plastic food packaging encourages obesity'.

Of course, this kind of packaging has benefits: such as giving food protection from temperature changes and as a barrier against air and water; it helps to keep food clean and fresh and to extend its shelf life; the labelling provides consumer information; and it provides an easy way of distributing, stocking, displaying and selling food. It has the further benefit of helping to control portion sizes, but there are downsides.

Packaged food that is prepared and ready to eat allows us to eat quickly and on the move, which is a sure-fire recipe for overeating. Packaged food also tends to be more energy dense. And there is evidence that the hormone-disrupting chemicals widely used today as plasticisers and stabilisers in the manufacture of food packaging – such as cellophane and bisphenol A (often used to line food tins) – may also contribute to the development of obesity.[1]

Interestingly, France uses less plastic food packaging than the UK and the US. And, guess what? France is near the bottom of the European obesity league table, with less than half the rate of obesity in the UK. It's also worth bearing in mind that the French have a completely different food culture from that of the UK and US. They eat real food that is properly prepared in the home, and they enjoy their food, usually spending time over their meals. Even though the food is often rich, their portions are small, and I'll be discussing portions later in this book. There is also a cultural norm in France that people shouldn't get fat, so women, especially, do control what they eat – and I'll be talking about having control over eating later.

The nature argument (or, it's all to do with our genes)

In contrast to Professor Wilding, Timothy Frayling, professor of human genetics at the University of Exeter, argued that it is genetic factors that decide who gets fat.

To try to explain why many people remain slim while others gain weight, he points out that genetic variation influences our appetites, metabolism and tolerance of physical activity. An analogy can be made with smoking: if everyone inhaled the same amount of cigarette smoke every day, the strongest risk factor for lung cancer would be genetic susceptibility to the adverse effects of cigarette smoke. If we were all to be exposed to the same amount of cigarette smoke, there would be enormous differences in how many of us would develop lung cancer and how many would not, and this can be explained only by genetic factors.

Twin and adoption studies show that variations in BMI (explained on pages 15–18) have a strong genetic component. One study assessed the heritability of BMI in over 20,000 young adult twin pairs from eight European countries. The correlation of BMI between identical twins was consistently stronger than that between non-identical same-sex twins. The estimated genetic effects, correcting for age and sex differences, were 60–70 per cent. In adoption studies with several hundred parent–biological child and parent–adoptee comparisons, children's BMI was consistently more strongly correlated with that of their biological parents than of their adoptive parents.[2]

In a study of over 5,000 twin pairs born in the UK during 1994–7, the correlation of BMI at ages eight to 11 years between identical twins was stronger than that between non-identical same-sex twins. The genetic effects were estimated as 77 per cent. Another study of over 2,000 very young twin pairs found that appetite had a genetic component. Correlations between appetite measures in one twin and weight of the other twin were stronger in identical than non-identical twin pairs.[3]

OK, it's true that twin studies may overestimate genetic effects, because there is less variation in the environment between children raised in the same household, and parents may treat identical twins differently to same-sex non-identical twins. But these factors are unlikely to explain the large differences in correlations of BMI between identical and non-identical twins.

Professor Frayling's conclusion is that genetic factors greatly influence our BMI, and research suggests that these genetic factors may operate largely through appetite control.

The bottom line

Recent research has shown that there is a genetic flaw, which greatly increases the risk of obesity in one in six people. The flaw is to do with a version of the FTO gene – the obesity or fat gene. This flawed, or high-risk, FTO gene changes levels of the hunger hormone, ghrelin, and makes fatty foods more tempting.

There is a strong family link with obesity, and our genes almost certainly play a major role in the risk of our becoming overweight.

We all have two copies of the FTO gene – one from each parent – and each copy comes in either a high-risk or a low-risk form. Those of us with two high-risk copies of the FTO gene are thought to be 70 per cent more likely to become obese than those with low-risk genes.

Going back to the debate in the BMJ, there followed a very vigorous exchange of views from a wide variety of doctors and health professionals, which underlines how far we are from any agreement as to why we become overweight and obese. But one fact is inescapable: evolution has caused us to become adapted to living in a different age, an age when food was scarce and it made sense to grab as much as we could, whenever we could. And it is likely to be hundreds, if not thousands, of years before our biology changes to a helpful one, if ever.

The predominant cause

My view, after studying the arguments and the enormous amount of feedback from health professionals in the *BMJ*, is that heredity and genetics account for over 75 per cent of obesity while environmental factors make up less than 25 per cent. People may be genetically predisposed to put on weight, and combined with the easily available packaged junk food, and decreased exercise, this makes it more likely that they will get fatter. Added to which, the plastics in convenience food might also have a role to play in why people who eat such food are more likely to put on weight. Bearing in mind that the obesity epidemic also links up with the dietary advice to eat low fat and more carbs, we also have increased amounts of foods containing sugar, which many people are eating because they think they are healthy.

So where does this leave us?

THE BODY-FAT STAT

For years we've all heard the advice: eat less and exercise more. We've been told that's the way to lose weight – but is that advice correct?

In theory, it should be, but in reality this advice has had precious little effect on our weight. We're more overweight, more obese than ever before. Even thin people are heavier than they were, say, 20 years ago. We are eating more now than we did, say, 30 years ago. The question is:

Why are we eating more?
Is it just greed, gluttony? Or is there more to it?

Clearly, there is far more to the subject than that. It seems that it has become harder to eat less, so why might this be? The answer is that it's all to do with something called the body-fat setpoint.

The body-fat setpoint

Our body has a complex mechanism to control how much fat we store – called our body-fat mass. Think of a room thermostat for the central heating. If the temperature drops too low, the boiler will kick in to deliver more heat. If the temperature rises too high, the boiler will cut out and, if you have an air-conditioning unit, this will kick in. It's the same with body fat. If food intake goes down, the body loses fat, but as soon as food intake goes up again, so body fat increases to its original level. Our body has a weight to which it always returns and at which point most of us seem to stay, regardless of any conscious effort to eat less or more. Think of it as our *default weight*.

The reason we always seem to revert to more or less the same weight without conscious effort is because of a feedback mechanism that results in an increase or decrease in fat mass in order to stabilise it. And it's because of this feedback, which always tries to maintain the same body fat, that just eating less doesn't work. Unless we remove whatever it is that's making our body want to store more fat, our body will continue to store fat even though we're not consuming the calories we need to continue storing fat. The feedback mechanism results in increased hunger, reduced metabolic rate and decreased body temperature. It also increases the efficiency of muscle contractions – in other words, our muscles do the same amount of work but use up less energy. And the result? Our fat mass increases to its previous level. Yes, we lose weight if we eat less, but the result is short-term, because our body fights to restore the lost fat – our body constantly defends its body-fat setpoint. The only way to control body weight in the long term is by *changing the setpoint* – which I like to call our body-fat stat.

IS EXERCISE THE ANSWER?

If we can't control our weight efficiently by a conscious effort to eat less, what about taking exercise? If we take more exercise, wouldn't that solve the problem?

On the face of it, this would seem to be the logical answer. But here's the glitch. We take more exercise to get rid of energy stored in our body (as fat), and look what happens: the fat stat kicks in. It sees all the energy leaving our body, and it registers that we have to replace it. And how does it do that? Hunger is the most obvious mechanism. After exercise, many of us feel more hungry, so we eat more in order to replace the calories we've just lost. Of course, exercise is great for fitness and it probably helps prevent us from becoming overweight in the first place. But, as a means of controlling weight, walking or jogging or running on a tread-mill is not as effective as many people think. Yes, of course, it helps – but just a little, not a lot.

In 2012, research at the University of Kansas was made over 16 months on both men and women. Each individual did 45 minutes of exercise, mainly on a treadmill, five days a week. Energy burned up was around 400 calories each session – far more than most people burn off in their weight-control exercise programmes. (Note: all calories in the book refer to kcals – kilocalories.) Almost half the men and women dropped out before the end of the 16-month period. And the results? The women maintained their baseline weight, BMI and fat mass –

they didn't lose any weight or body fat. By contrast, men lost an average of 11 pounds (5kg). This may sound quite a lot, but it is on average just 2½ ounces (72g) a week! Another way of looking at it is that it took on average three months for men to lose just 2¼ pounds (1kg).[4] Here's another thought. What do many of us do after exercise? We think how good we've been and we reward ourselves – with food, which is often rich in carbs! (I'll be discussing the different kinds of carbs later in this chapter and in Chapter 8.)

For losing weight, the only way exercise *traditionally* helps is if we do a lot of it and we don't reward ourselves afterwards with food. But now there is a different way: high-intensity interval training (HIIT). And that's what we'll be focusing on later in this book. Of course, it's still important that we don't reward ourselves afterwards with food – but the temptation is far smaller following HIIT compared with traditional exercise.

To maintain weight once we've got down to our target figure, regular exercise does seem to be helpful. And, of course, exercise, including HIIT, is so beneficial for our health.

WE NEED TO FOCUS ON OUR EATING

The next question is:

Should we focus on calories or carbohydrates?

This is the big debate – but there is no agreement. The 'calories in/calories out' theory is that losing weight is simply a matter of burning off more calories than those we consume, regardless of the food type. But some people believe that restricting calories by restricting carbs is more effective than simply restricting calories regardless of food type.

Is a low-carb diet, then, the answer? Interestingly, research shows that when people are allowed to eat as much as they like while following either a low-carb or a low-fat diet, the low-carb dieters eat fewer calories. Why is this? It may be that the low-carb diet triggers biological processes that result in resetting the fat stat. That sounds a wonderful solution. Or is it? Do we really want to be on a low-carb diet for the rest of our lives? Because research shows that even if we lose weight on a low-carb diet and reset our fat stat, going back to our old ways of eating results in the fat stat being reset upwards and weight piling on again.

If a low-carb diet isn't the long-term solution, what else should we think about?

THE ROLE OF GUT FLORA IN WEIGHT CONTROL

Recently, research has focused on the bacteria that live in our gut, called our gut flora. Gut bacteria have a crucial role in nutrition and health. They are important in synthesising vitamins. Changes to the gut flora are also linked to obesity and type-2 diabetes. Laboratory mice that have no bacteria in their gut do not become obese when overfed, whereas other mice with normal bacteria in their gut become obese when overfed.

Gut flora powerfully influences our body-fat mass. When scientists take gut flora from obese mice and put it into bacteria-free lean mice, guess what happens? The lean mice become obese.[5]

We don't yet know precisely why this happens. It may be that the 'bad' bacteria stimulate an increase in appetite, so the mice end up eating more. And it's possible that the same happens in humans. But there's probably more to it than that. It's probable that good or bad bacteria affect our metabolism and hormones, and this makes it more or less likely that we gain weight. In Chapter 4 I'll be discussing gut flora further and how to nurture yours.

THE HUNGER HORMONE – LEPTIN

As we've already seen, our body-fat mass secretes a hormone called leptin. The amount of leptin is directly proportional to the amount of our body fat. Leptin acts as a signal to a part of our brain called the hypothalamus to let it know how much fat we have and to suppress appetite when we have sufficient. The more fat we have, the more leptin will be signalled to the brain to take appropriate action: increase metabolism, decrease hunger, and so on.

This system can go wrong, however. The hypothalamus fails to respond as it should to leptin and it becomes increasingly resistant to it. This happens for several reasons. Probably the most important is that the hypothalamus becomes inflamed, most likely because gut flora cause a low-grade inflammation that spreads to the brain.

There are several other reasons, all quite complicated, why leptin resistance happens, but the point is that as we gain fat leptin signals the hypothalamus to decrease our hunger and increase our activity levels to maintain the fat stat. As time goes on and more fat is deposited, more and more leptin has to be produced for the hypothalamus to react – thereby creating leptin resistance – while the hypothalamus continually fails to do its job in regulating our body weight correctly.

How leptin's efficiency can be disrupted

Leptin can also be affected by *lectins* from the foods we eat, making it inefficient. Lectins are large protein molecules that are present in most plants and which are able to bind to the complex sugar molecules that make up much of the surface of every cell of every living organism. They enable animal and plant cells to communicate with each other.

Plants use them as a defence mechanism against animals – to avoid being eaten. A prime example is raw kidney beans. The beans' lectins bind to the sugar molecules on the surface of our red blood cells. This makes the red blood cells clump together, which makes our blood clot – therefore killing us! It takes only five raw beans to do this.

Kidney beans are not the most poisonous vegetable to humans, however. The castor bean contains ricin, a powerful lectin that is one of the deadliest of all poisons (and popular as a biological weapon). One single molecule, inhaled or injected, is instantly fatal.

Lectins are toxic and inflammatory, and are able to interfere with our body's communication system. This is very significant when we consider how insulin and leptins work in our body. Insulin (see Chapter 8) is the fat-storage hormone. It binds to a receptor on each fat cell, making the fat cell take up (ingest) or make more fat. Once insulin has played its part, it detaches from the fat cell and moves on, thus preventing too much fat being deposited. The problem arises if we eat potatoes, wheat, lentils, green peas and corn. These foods contain lectins, which attach to the same insulin receptor on fat cells. Then trouble is, unlike insulin, once lectin becomes attached it never detaches. The result is that the fat cell continues to store more and more fat.

'But hold on!' you say. When fat cells are full, don't they manufacture the hormone leptin, and doesn't leptin go to our brain to tell it we're full and we should stop eating? Absolutely. The problem is that those fiendish lectins, not content with binding to our fat cells, also bind to the receptor sites for leptin in the brain, which of course blocks its effect on satiety. The more lectins we eat, the hungrier we get!

So we need to know which foods are highest in lectins so that we can minimise them. They are:

▶ All grains – especially wheat and wheatgerm, quinoa, buckwheat, oats, barley, rye and corn

▶ Pulses – especially dried beans, including soya and peanuts

▶ Nuts

▶ Dairy (cow's and goat's)

▶ Nightshades – potatoes, peppers, tomatoes, aubergine, chillies

▶ Oils made from the above foods

Of course, I'm not saying we should *always* avoid foods high in lectins. My advice is to eat them in moderation. For this reason, you will find some of them in the recipes in this book.

Which foods are low in lectins? These include:

▶ Carrots, asparagus, mushrooms, onions, cauliflower, leafy greens, broccoli, pak choi, squash, sweet potatoes, yams

▶ Berries, cherries, citrus fruits, apples, pineapple

▶ Fish and seafood

▶ Meat and poultry

▶ Eggs

WHAT ABOUT CARBS?

Carbs are a whole chapter on their own, so we'll look at them in much more detail later in the book. But, for now, the important point is this: there's a huge difference between refined and unrefined carbohydrates. If we eat unrefined – that is, whole-food carbohydrates – we encourage the growth of good bacteria, which feed on the fibre in whole-food carbs. Refined carbs – such as white flour and sugar – on the other hand, encourage bad bacteria at the expense of the good ones. In the 1950s, the incidence of obesity was low even though the consumption of carbs was high – and that's because very few of the carbs we ate were refined.

A BALANCING ACT: OMEGA-3 AND OMEGA-6 ESSENTIAL FATS

Omega-3 and omega-6 fats are known as 'essential' because the body must take them from food. Omega-6 is the polyunsaturated fat found mainly in seed oils such as corn oil, safflower oil and soya oil (sold as vegetable oil). Our consumption of these oils has increased dramatically over the years. The typical Western diet today contains poly- and monounsaturated margarine, as well as cooking and salad oils, and these provide large amounts of fats, especially omega-6 fatty acids. Omega-3 oils are found predominantly in oily fish and grass-fed meat, such as lamb. The balance between the omega-6 and omega-3 fats determines how our body reacts to harmful stimuli. Omega-6 oils are inflammatory, and therefore too much of this in the body increases inflammation. When this happens in our brain, leptin resistance increases. The result is that we become overweight and find it difficult to lose weight.

In primitive societies, when we were hunter-gatherers, we humans consumed omega-3s and omega-6s in more or less the same amounts. But in modern times the amount of omega-6s in the diet may be as much as 20 times that of omega-3s.

If we want to lose weight, we need to look at our consumption of omega-3s and omega-6s. This is not to say that increasing omega-3s and reducing omega-6s is going to bring about a dramatic and rapid weight loss – more's the pity! – but it should be part of our long-term approach for weight control.

Patients ask me: is it OK to use seed oils? My answer is, yes, but in very small amounts in cooking. In fact, these oils are often more practical for high cooking temperatures than, say, olive oil, which is more suitable for using in salads.

Now that we have this knowledge we can look more deeply into ways to control weight gain and encourage weight loss.

Part Two

LET'S THINK STRATEGIES

Chapter Four

HOW TO PREVENT WEIGHT GAIN AND HELP WEIGHT LOSS

I N THIS CHAPTER I'LL EXPLAIN how the key to losing weight, and preventing weight gain, is to focus on the correct areas – that is, the effective amounts of exercise, plus eating food that will nourish you and protect your gut – instead of becoming bogged down in the idea that you must be exercising more and more and eating less and less.

RETHINKING EXERCISE

Earlier I explained that traditional long or stamina exercise, such as spending 20–25 minutes walking or in a gym two to three times a week, results in fairly modest weight-loss benefits, and often the results can be disappointing. On the other hand, high-intensity interval training (HIIT) offers real benefits.

Scientists don't yet fully understand why high-intensity training can help weight loss. One thing is certain: it isn't to do with calories. After all, how many calories can you burn off in a minute or two? Not many. We do know, however, that exercise reduces inflammation in our body – and that includes our hypothalamus, which increases leptin sensitivity, thereby telling our body that it has enough fat. HIIT also improves *insulin sensitivity* – and that's important because *decreasing* insulin sensitivity is linked to weight gain, as I will explain in Chapter 8.

Earlier, I explained how moderate exercise, such as jogging, makes us use 40 per cent of our muscles, whereas HIIT exercise uses 80 per cent of our muscles. This means that more glycogen (the stored sugar in our muscles) is broken down. Research suggests that at least four out of five us – that's 80 per cent – would benefit from HIIT exercise.

As with moderate exercise, we're not talking about huge weight losses – so adjusting how we eat still remains most important – but the benefits for 80 per cent of us are certainly worthwhile.

The major reason that people give for not exercising is time, so the brevity of HIIT will appeal to many of us who want to lose weight.

Incidentally, only healthy exercisers should participate in HIIT workouts, as these extreme bouts of physical activity increase the risk of injury and burnout. If you are in any doubt as to your suitability or if you are taking any medications, it's very important to consult your doctor first.

HIIT – is this really so fantastic for weight loss?

I think most of us would be highly sceptical of claims that very short bursts of intense physical activity could make long, boring exercise redundant, so let's look at the research.

Dr Stephen Boutcher, of the University of New South Wales, Australia, has a special interest in this area. He suggests from his research that HIIT can result in reductions in subcutaneous fat (the fat immediately under the skin) and abdominal body fat in young, normal-weight people and in those who are slightly over-weight. He thinks it's probably to do with HIIT increasing fat oxidation during and after exercise and also that it suppresses the appetite. (Fat oxidation is the breaking down in the body of large fat molecules into smaller molecules that it can use for energy.) It is known that regular HIIT increases both aerobic and anaer-obic fitness and it also lowers insulin resistance and increases our muscles' capacity to oxidise fatty acids. Aerobic fitness is the abil-ity to walk or do other exercise for long periods of time. Regular aerobic exercise makes for a healthier heart. Anaerobic fitness, which is the result of resistance training, helps strengthen mus-cles. Insulin resistance is the condition in which the body's cells fail to respond to the normal actions of the hormone insulin, and this eventually leads to type-2 diabetes.

What's the best kind of HIIT for weight loss?

Insulin resistance has recently been shown to be mainly located in leg muscle, and because HIIT exercise focuses on the legs – such as cycling and the many workouts described later in this book – it is likely that these areas will show the greatest increase in insulin sensitivity, with loss of both subcutaneous and abdom-inal fat. Because insulin encourages the laying down of fat in the body, the more efficiently the body's cells respond to insulin – that is, the greater the sensitivity to insulin – the less fat will be deposited. The parts of the body where cells seem to respond best to insulin are in the large leg muscles, and because HIIT con-centrates mainly on the legs, this type of exercise can be extremely efficient for fat loss.

LOOKING AT DIET

Around the world there are cultures in which virtually no one becomes fat. What are they eating that's different to what many of us are eating in the UK, US, Australia and a growing number of countries around the world? The answer is whole foods, both animal and plant foods, all rich in nutrients and traditionally prepared. These people don't develop the metabolic diseases we see in our society and they don't become overweight – until they adopt Western foods, and then they become like many of us: overweight, obese, diabetic, and so on.

We must surely ask what's so different about those healthy societies' whole-food diets compared to our own? There are several differences, but the most important one is this: they don't eat refined sugar, whereas we do. Nor do those societies eat white flour. Nor do they consume our modern industrial seed oils, such as corn oil and soya.

Of course, the healthy diets of those healthy societies contain *no processed food*, which is made up of too many refined carbs and not enough fibre.

There is one other aspect of diet that we need to consider: food sensitivities. These can contribute to increased body-fat mass. Many of us will know people who, for example, stop eating wheat and lose dramatic amounts of weight. Wheat contains gluten, which is also present rye and barley, so gluten-sensitive people need to avoid those grains as well. Another fairly common food sensitivity, which can contribute to obesity, is milk and dairy products. Giving up wheat and/or dairy for a week or two to see if symptoms improve is well worth a try.

IMPROVING YOUR GUT FLORA –
PREBIOTICS AND PROBIOTICS

Prebiotics and probiotics are very much the buzzwords in health today, but what's the difference between the two?

Prebiotics are fermented food ingredients that promote beneficial changes in our gut flora that are good for our overall health. There are many prebiotic foods, but there are two that we particularly know about: oligosaccharides and inulin. The best natural food sources of these include raw chicory root, raw Jerusalem artichoke, raw garlic, raw leek, raw or cooked onion, raw asparagus, raw wheat bran, cooked wholewheat flour, and raw banana. (Chicory root is usually consumed either as a coffee substitute or as a dietary supplement or food additive.)

Probiotics are live bacteria that are good for our health. The two commonest groups of probiotics are lactic acid bacteria (LAB) and bifidobacteria. They are present in fermented foods with specially added active live cultures, such as in yogurt, or as dietary supplements. Probiotics increase the ability of the gut, especially the lower bowel, known as the large bowel, to keep inflammatory molecules out of the blood. Remember, if you keep inflammatory molecules out of the blood and away from the brain, the brain becomes more sensitive to leptin, which in turn helps weight control.

Probiotics can be beneficial in so many ways that doctors often advise them for patients with certain health problems, such as *Candida* and irritable-bowel syndrome. There are many probiotic supplements and drinks available in supermarkets; however, my favourites are Symprove and VSL#3. These contain live bacteria, rather than freeze-dried ones, which undoubtedly accounts for their superior benefits over most other probiotics. They are most easily available online.

WEIGHT-LOSS STRATEGIES

We've looked at various factors that affect whether or not we become overweight, but how can we use these to help reduce weight when we've already become overweight and raised our fat stat?

We'll look at these in more detail in later chapters, but for now the message is clear: don't focus on cutting calories or doing endless workouts in the gym. Instead, focus on improving your immune system and reducing inflammation in the body. As well as helping you to lose weight, this will improve your health and well-being.

This book will demonstrate how easy it is to make small, subtle changes to your diet that will achieve that result. Those changes won't require you to drastically change what you eat.

At the same time, however, small changes to your level of physical activity in the form of HIIT, combined with these small changes in your diet, can produce really amazing results for weight loss.

Chapter Five

DODGING THE MINEFIELDS

SOME OBSTACLES TO LOSING weight can be devastating, which is why I call them minefields. Having strategies to avoid them will help with your success.

THE MINEFIELDS

Let's look at a few of the common minefields you might encounter.

The all-or-nothing approach

There is a common all-or-nothing mindset that says, 'I've eaten something I shouldn't have done. I've messed up, so I might as well give up.' Or, 'I haven't exercised for two days. Ah well, I might as well not bother.'

Have you watched a professional skater fall in a skating competition? What does she or he do? They get up and continue the routine as though nothing had happened.

One mistake doesn't blow it all. We all have slip-ups. The trick is to get on regardless.

Low self-esteem

It's so easy to put life on hold until we've reached our target weight, saying to ourselves that we don't have any self-worth until we've shed all those excess pounds. This mindset becomes an unbearable weight. The trick is to visualise ourselves looking the way we imagine we will when we had achieved our goals, and then to live as if we had already achieved those goals. This is such a powerful positive for our minds and it works far better than holding on to low self-esteem.

Confusing physical and emotional hunger

Many of us confuse physical and emotional hunger. A good way to deal with this is to keep an eating diary. Write down *everything* you eat and drink, including when and how you felt at the time. Most importantly, write down if you are hungry at the time. You'll find it very revealing.

Inappropriate eating behaviour

Feeling the need to eat can be prompted by many things that aren't actually to do with hunger. (See also Chapter 15, where I give you some hints on eating mindfully.)

Not taking enough physical activity

Although this might appear self-evident, physical activity is not just about going as hard as you can at the gym for an hour. It's no surprise that many people don't fancy doing this. Physical activity is about moving around as much as possible during the day, rather than sitting for long periods, plus taking yourself off for a walk for 30 minutes to get your whole body moving. An active day will make you feel less inclined to nibble on snacks out of boredom, because moving about gives us a feeling of well-being.

The effects of dehydration

It's so easy to confuse dehydration with hunger. That's why it's important to drink plenty of low-calorie, non-caffeine and non-alcoholic drinks. The old idea of eight glasses a day has been somewhat discredited. My advice now is to make sure you drink plenty of fluids, sufficient to ensure that you aren't thirsty.

HOW TO COMBAT THE MINEFIELDS

Losing weight is simple – but it's not always easy. Most of us know what to do, but sticking to our plan can often be a huge challenge. Things can go swimmingly for a time and then suddenly we become unstuck. It's going to happen, so the best thing is to accept it – and to have a strategy in place. Here are a few strategies that many people find helpful.

Be positive

Adopt a positive attitude to losing weight. Try to think of losing weight as a positive experience. That's going to be hard to do if you have a tough and demanding diet, which is why following an approach, like this one, that doesn't require superhuman amounts of willpower is so important.

Be realistic

Set a realistic weight-loss goal. If you've a lot of weight to lose, break it up into smaller manageable chunks; for example, if you ultimately want to lose, say, 1 stone 12 pounds (12kg), set yourself an initial target of, say, about 9 pounds (4kg), and focus on that. Alcoholics talk about thinking of just one day at a time; with weight loss it's a good idea to think of 2¼ pounds (1kg) at a time.

Make behavioural changes

As well as focusing on small weight changes, focus more on behavioural changes than on the weight changes. It will give you an insight into what you can change to make your weight loss achievements easier. Are you munching away while watching television, for example? The chances are that you're not even hungry – it's just something you're used to doing. It's specific actions that lead to weight gain and loss. Recognising these will help you.

Ask yourself why you failed last time you tried to lose weight or what happened the last time the weight you'd shed made an unwelcome return. Was it a poor diet? Or lack of support from family members? Try to ensure the same doesn't happen again.

Make small changes in your lifestyle. If you're used to eating out several times a week – whether it's in restaurants or at friends' homes – don't suddenly stop it completely. Cut down a little and, when you are eating away from home, try to control what you eat and, most importantly, how much you eat.

Know that there will be setbacks

Setbacks happen – accept that truth. It's a fact of life. But be like the professional skater who falls: get up and continue where you left off.

Don't be outwitted by nutrition labels

Labels on foods can be another minefield. We'll look at how to read them in Chapter 10 on Smart Fats, Unsmart Fats.

GET THE RIGHT MINDSET FOR BEING FULLY PREPARED

An important reason why some people fail in their weight-loss programme is that they're not fully prepared. They haven't thought the process through. Here are some vital issues that we all need to think about before embarking on weight loss, which, as I've already said, is very simple but often far from easy.

Have the right attitude

Losing weight isn't just about getting your figure into good shape for the summer holiday. Of course, that's a good initial incentive, but it's vital to remain motivated in the long term. Overweight and obesity are chronic conditions. This means that the tendency to put on weight never goes away. We can't cure it in the sense that once we've lost the weight it just stays off automatically. We have to work at it and control it, permanently. Unfortunately, many of us give up when we don't see quick results. And yet, slow weight loss is much more likely to be permanent weight loss.

Change your lifestyle

Losing weight isn't about dieting – it's about *lifestyle*. Small changes to our food choices and physical activity can permanently influence our weight – and *permanently* is the key to successful weight control. If we want to lose weight and lead a healthier life, we need to change the way we live. This doesn't require any overnight transformations, but periodically finding new ways of doing things is highly recommended. Some of the ways that others have found success in changing their lifestyle include concentrating on their daily routines, limitations, schedules and the food items that they surround themselves with, such as not having any crisps in their home.

Be more active

Continuing on from the point above about lifestyle, it's almost impossible to lose weight and to keep it off without a reasonable level of physical activity. I don't necessarily mean the gym, which, let's face it, is a glorified torture chamber for many of us. No, it's all about walking more, using the stairs instead of the lift, and so on. Do you have a downstairs toilet as well as one upstairs? How about using the one that's further away from you during the day? And then of course there is HIIT – more of that later in this book.

Eat smartly

Become familiar with healthy foods compared with unhealthy ones. Become expert at reading nutrition labels (see Chapter 10). Remember that portions are important – size matters! Think about keeping an eating diary (see page 176) – it's amazing how much less food many of us eat if we have to write everything down. See pages 232–5 to help you with portion sizes.

Cultivate a support system

Having the support of your family can be enormously helpful, especially if they eat the same food as you do. Having a friend we can call when things get tough or simply to exchange ideas or even to work out together – a slim-buddy – is really good.

Understand your own biology

The more we have to lose, the faster the weight will go, but, as we lose weight, the rate of further weight loss inevitably slows down. This is because losing body fat reduces our metabolic rate, and the slower our metabolism becomes, the slower our weight loss will be. Also, as we've already seen, our body fights to protect our fat.

Address the issues that you *can* change

Of course, reduced metabolic rate is not the only reason why some of us fail to lose weight, but, although it's just about the only one we can do little about, we can certainly do a *lot* about the other reasons, such as:

▶ **Falling off the wagon** Of course, we can all fall off the wagon occasionally – Christmas, barbecues, a restaurant, supper with friends – but is it really just occasionally, or is it becoming a regular habit?

▶ **Portion creep** Are your portion sizes still as small as when you started on your weight-loss programme – or have they started to creep up?

▶ **Weekends and holidays** These are the times when we change our daily routines. But we need to be careful we don't change our eating and physical activity routines other than very occasionally.

▶ **Losing patience** Losing weight successfully and permanently entails losing weight *slowly*. Rapid weight loss is almost always followed by weight *regain*. Some of us become so frustrated at how slowly our weight comes off that we become discouraged and then we give up. To use the cliché, Rome wasn't built in a day!

▶ **Eating behaviour** If this doesn't change, our weight won't change. It's as simple as that. And there's lots about eating behaviour later in this book.

Finally, as I've said many times in this book, remember three key points:

1 Overweight and obesity are long-term conditions. We cannot cure them – we can only control them.

2 In order to control them permanently, we need a sustainable approach. This means lifestyle changes, not a diet.

3 Losing weight, and keeping it off, is simple – but it's not easy. In order to succeed, we have to be, and remain, absolutely committed to the process. It's about determination. It's about visualising and feeling how we'll look and feel when we reach our target weight.

Part Three

THE 12-MINUTE EXERCISE PROGRAMME

Chapter Six

AN INTRODUCTION TO HIIT

A S I HAVE MENTIONED EARLIER, the principle of high-intensity interval training (HIIT) is that the exercise uses 80 per cent of your body muscles. Traditional non-HIIT exercise uses only 40 per cent, so HIIT uses as many muscles in your body as possible and at the same time pushes your heart rate to the maximum. It's such a successful form of training that it's incorporated into the training programmes of almost all athletes today.

Not all exercises are suitable for everyone, however. Before attempting a new exercise regime consider your overall health, strength and flexibility to see if a particular exercise is suitable for you. Remember, almost any exercise can result in personal injury. **If you have any doubts as to your fitness to carry out an exercise, please consult your doctor first**.

The aim of the 12-Minute Weight-Loss Plan is to achieve fat burning in just 12 minutes *a week*. This is split into three 4-minute sessions, each session separated by at least 48 hours. It is neither necessary nor desirable to exercise on consecutive days, since the benefits of HIIT carry over for two to three days and your body needs 48 hours to recover after each session.

THE HIIT SESSIONS

My HIIT regimen is based on the one invented by Professor Izumi Tabata for helping Japanese Olympic skaters to achieve maximum fitness. His original session consists of 20 seconds of ultra-intense exercise followed by 10 seconds of rest, repeated continuously for 4 minutes. In this book there is a small variation on this: the first 30 seconds and the last 30 seconds are warm-up and cool-down periods. Each 4-minute session consists of:

  1 Warm-up: 30 seconds

  2 HIIT exercise no. 1: 20 seconds

  3 Gentle exercise: 10 seconds

  4 HIIT exercise no. 2: 20 seconds

  5 Gentle exercise: 10 seconds

  6 HIIT exercise no. 3: 20 seconds

  7 Gentle exercise: 10 seconds

  8 HIIT exercise no. 4: 20 seconds

  9 Gentle exercise: 10 seconds

10 HIIT exercise no. 5: 20 seconds

11 Gentle exercise: 10 seconds

12 HIIT exercise no. 6: 20 seconds

13 Gentle exercise: 10 seconds

14 Cool-down: 30 seconds

As time goes by, and you become fitter, you may want to lengthen your exercise time to five minutes, which amounts to 15 minutes a week. Most people, even those who hate the idea of exercise, won't find this too much of a task. Each 5-minute programme would consist of:

1 Warm-up: 30 seconds

2 HIIT exercise no. 1: 20 seconds

3 Gentle exercise: 10 seconds

4 HIIT exercise no. 2: 20 seconds

5 Gentle exercise: 10 seconds

6 HIIT exercise no. 3: 20 seconds

7 Gentle exercise: 10 seconds

8 HIIT exercise no. 4: 20 seconds

9 Gentle exercise: 10 seconds

10 HIIT exercise no. 5: 20 seconds

11 Gentle exercise: 10 seconds

12 HIIT exercise no. 6: 20 seconds

13 Gentle exercise: 10 seconds

14 HIIT exercise no. 7: 20 seconds

15 Gentle exercise: 10 seconds

16 HIIT exercise no. 8: 20 seconds

17 Gentle exercise: 10 seconds

18 Cool-down: 30 seconds

TIP

An easy way to time yourself in the different steps of the programme is by using a smartphone interval timer app, such as a Tabata timer. There are several free ones available to download from the internet, and you can program them to provide your own custom timings.

THE WARM-UP AND COOL-DOWN

Warming up your muscles before you exercise is important. You will increase the temperature and flexibility of your muscles and be more efficient and safer during your workout. A typical warm-up might be gentle jogging on the spot, getting your heels up as close as you can to your bottom. Use your entire body: as you jog, move your arms around as much as possible. Another warm-up is to cross your arms over your chest and do 10 easy squats. Don't skip the warm-up, otherwise you will risk injury and poor performance. Fortunately, as HIIT is of such short duration, you need only a short warm-up and cool-down.

The cool-down after your workout is just as important as the warm-up. After working out, your heart rate is high, your body temperature is higher, and your blood vessels are dilated, so, if you stop too fast, you could feel sick or even faint. To cool down, do gentle jogging on the spot or walking. Try also to stretch your leg muscles.

YOUR HEART RATE

The aim of HIIT is to push your heart rate to close to its maximum, but what is your maximum heart rate? This will vary with age. There are many different ways of calculating maximum heart rate. A popular one, used by many fitness trainers and fitness assessors, is the one I use. It's is a simple calculation:

$$220 - age$$

For example, if you are 30 years old, your maximum heart rate is 220 – 30 = 190. If you are 50 your maximum heart rate is 220 – 50 = 170.

When you first start doing HIIT, aim for a heart rate that is 70 per cent of your maximum heart rate. Eventually, as you become fitter, you can speed up to 85 per cent of maximum heart rate.

Once fit:

For a 30-year-old this is 190 × 0.85 = 162 approx.

For a 50-year-old this is 170 × 0.85 = 145 approx.

For a 70-year-old it is 150 × 0.85 =128 approx.

Below is a table showing:

▶ The maximum heart rate (MHR) at each age.

▶ 70 per cent MHR, which is a good starting point if you're not very fit.

▶ 85 per cent MHR, which is the heart rate to aim for eventually when you've become fitter.

MAXIMUM HEART-RATE LEVELS

Age	MHR	70% of MHR	85% of MHR
20	200	140	170
25	195	137	166
30	190	133	162
35	185	130	157
40	180	126	153
45	175	123	149
50	170	119	145
55	165	116	140
60	160	112	136
65	155	109	132
70	150	105	128
75	145	102	123
80	140	98	119

How to measure your heart rate

Measure your pulse rate (at your wrist or at the side of your neck) for six seconds, then multiply that number by 10; for example, if there are seven beats in six seconds, this means your heart rate is 7 × 10 = 70 per minute. Another way is to buy a simple heart-rate monitor.

You may be asking, 'How do I know HIIT works? How do I know it can help me to lose weight?' These are very good questions, and you will find some of the evidence in Appendix 1.

Chapter Seven

THE HIIT EXERCISES

THERE ARE MANY DIFFERENT WAYS of performing HIIT. The exercises can be done indoors or outdoors, in a gym or in your home, with equipment or without. Each has its devotees and others who hate that type and prefer something else. Personally, I don't like gyms and I'm not keen on machines, so I prefer to do home-based or outdoor exercise. The exercises in this chapter do not require that you visit a gym, and need no machines. They fall into four main types:

1 Running

2 Cycling

3 Swimming

4 Stairs

Of course, there are many others, such as rowing, trampolining and boxing – the list is almost endless.

All the exercises involve the same basic pattern – 20 seconds of intense physical activity, followed by 10 seconds' rest or gentle exercise, repeated.

RUNNING

If you are out on a walk or a jog, run as fast as you can for 20 seconds (imagine you're running to catch the last bus home), raising your knees high and pumping your arms. Then slow down to a gentle jog for 10 seconds. Then get back into the run for 20 seconds, then slow jog for 10 seconds. Keep repeating this for four minutes.

CYCLING

While out cycling (or using an indoor static cycle), cycle as fast as you can for 20 seconds, then cycle gently for 10 seconds. Cycle as fast as you can for 20 seconds, then cycle gently for 10 seconds. Keep repeating this for four minutes.

SWIMMING

While swimming, swim as fast as you can for 20 seconds, then swim gently for 10 seconds. Swim as fast as you can for 20 seconds, then swim gently for 10 seconds. Keep repeating this for four minutes. If you're on your own, it may be difficult to time this, so you may prefer to measure by distance, such as two widths fast swim followed by one width slow swim.

STAIRS

This is a really great way to do HIIT, but you do need a staircase that goes up several floors. Run upstairs as fast as you can in 20 seconds, then walk on the spot for 10 seconds. Run upstairs as fast as you can in 20 seconds, then walk on the spot for 10 seconds. Keep repeating this for four minutes. Now you can see why you need a staircase that goes up many floors!

THE HIIT WORKOUTS

There are many, many different HIIT workouts. Below I've described 20 that are my favourites.

There are also many different ways you can use the workouts. Remember, depending on whether you decide your four-minute routine will include your warm-up and cool-down or not, you'll be doing six or eight high-intensity exercises, each lasting 20 seconds with 10 seconds' rest in between.

▶ **Option 1** Use the same workout for each of the 20-second activities.

▶ **Option 2** Alternate between two different workouts for each of the 20-second activities.

▶ **Option 3** Adopt a different workout for each and every 20-second activity.

The beauty of this approach is that you can vary your regimen as much as you like. In this way you can avoid the enemy of reluctant exercisers – boredom!

High knees

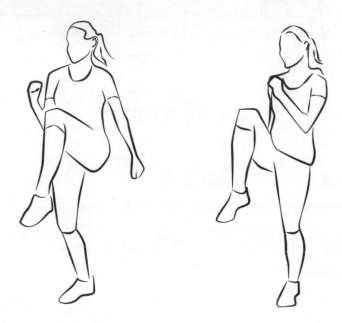

1. Run on one spot, bringing your knees up to your chest as high as you can. At the same time, pump your arms.

2. Do the exercise as fast as you can for 20 seconds.

3. In the standing position, do gentle running on the spot for 10 seconds.

4. Repeat the above.

ADVICE: try to bring your knees up as high as you can. Try to land on the balls of your feet as you run, and switch legs as fast as you can.

Burpees

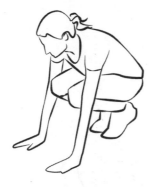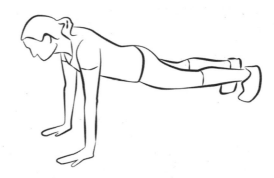

1. Stand upright.

2. Drop into a squat position, hands on the ground.

3. Keeping your arms extended, kick both your feet back.

4. Return your feet to the squat position.

5. Stand upright.

6. Do the exercise as fast as you can, with as many repeats as you can in 20 seconds.

7. In the standing position, do gentle running on the spot for 10 seconds.

8. Repeat the above.

Jump lunges

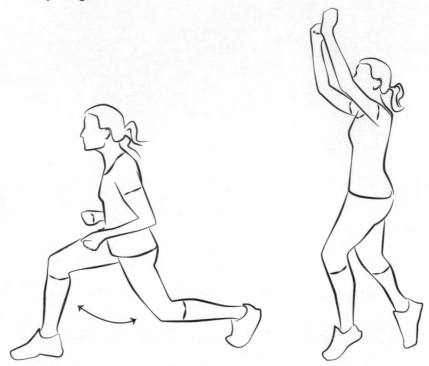

1. Stand with your feet together, elbows bent at 90 degrees.

2. Lunge forward with your right foot.

3. Jump straight up as you thrust your arms forward, keeping your knees bent.

4. Switch legs in midair, like a scissor action.

5. Land in a lunge with your left leg forward.

6. Repeat, switching legs again.

7. Repeat the above for 20 seconds.

8. In the standing position, do gentle running on the spot for 10 seconds.

9. Repeat the above.

Spiderman

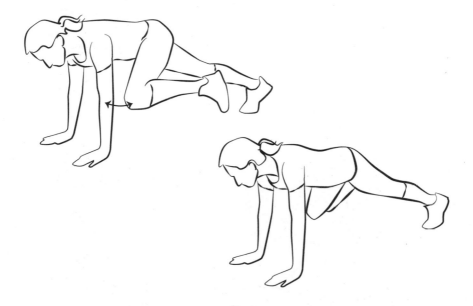

1. Start in the push-up position with your arms straight below you, hands on the ground, shoulder-width apart, your legs extended. Your body should form a straight line from head to heels.

2. Bring your right knee towards the your right elbow, then extend it straight behind you while at the same time bringing your left knee towards your left elbow, then extend the knee straight behind you as you bring your right knee again towards your right elbow, and so on.

3. Repeat the above for 20 seconds.

4. Rest for 10 seconds.

5. Repeat the above.

Deep squats

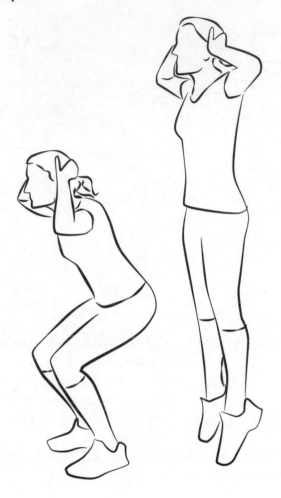

1. Stand with your legs shoulder-width apart and knees slightly bent.

2. Squat down as low as possible. Explosively push back up with your legs.

3. Repeat the above for 20 seconds.

4. Rest for 10 seconds.

5. Repeat the above.

Squat jacks

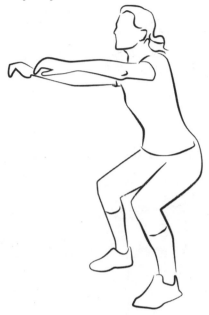 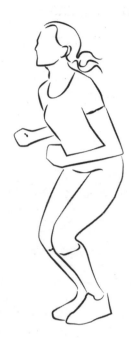

1. Lower yourself into the squat position and bring your arms in front of you.

2. Holding the squat position, jump your feet together. At the same time swing your arms back by your sides, keeping your elbows bent.

3. Keep 'jacking' your feet out and in as quickly as you can without coming up out of your squat.

4. Do this as fast as you can for 20 seconds.

5. Adopt the standing position and do gentle running on the spot for 10 seconds.

6. Repeat the above.

ADVICE Make sure you keep the squat position as you do the jacks by keeping your knees behind your toes and your hips behind you as if you were sitting in a chair.

Squat thrusts (a variation on burpees)

1. Stand with your feet shoulder-width apart, knees slightly bent.

2. Squat down, placing your hands about shoulder-width apart on the floor. (Don't go past 90 degrees at the knee; go to the point where you can reach the floor before you jump your legs back.)

3. Kick both your feet out behind you, which results in you being in a push-up position.

4. With your knees or feet on the floor, do a push-up while keeping your back straight.

5. Jump back to a squat position.

6. Stand upright.

7. In the standing position, do gentle running on the spot for 10 seconds.

8. Repeat the above.

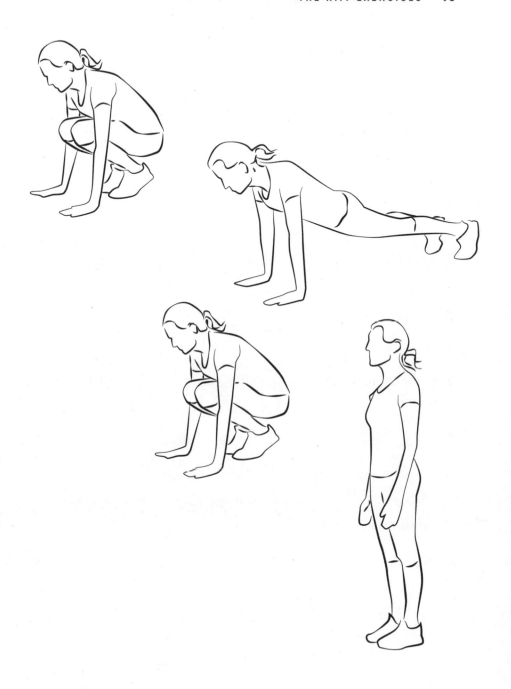

Jumping jacks

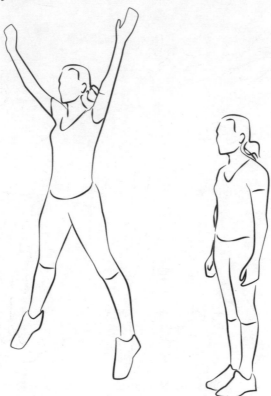

1. Stand on with your knees slightly bent.

2. Jump as high as you can, extending your arms and legs out to the side like a jumping jack.

3. Land with your feet just inside your shoulder width.

4. After you land, pull your arms and legs back together.

5. Do the exercise as fast as you can, with as many repeats as you can in 20 seconds.

6. Adopt the standing position and do gentle jogging on the spot for 10 seconds.

7. Repeat the above.

Vertical jacks (a variation on jumping jacks)

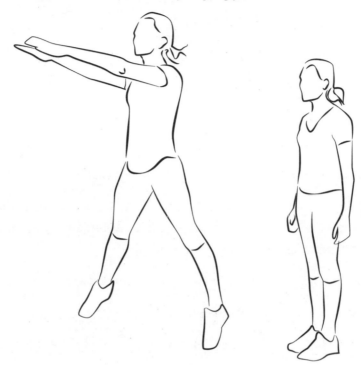

1. Stand with your knees slightly bent.

2. Jump as high as you can, extending your arms out in front of you and your legs out to the side.

3. Land with your feet just inside your shoulder width.

4. After you land, pull your arms and legs back together.

5. Do the exercise as fast as you can, with as many repeats as you can in 20 seconds.

6. Adopt the standing position and do gentle jogging on the spot for 10 seconds.

7. Repeat the above.

Up-and-out jacks (a variation on jumping jacks)

1. Stand with your knees slightly bent.

2. Squat down towards the ground.

3. Jump as high as you can, extending your arms and legs out to the side like a jumping jack.

4. Land with your feet just inside your shoulder width.

5. After you land, pull your arms and legs back together.

6. Jump as high as you can, this time extending your arms so that your hands come up in front of your body and over your head instead of sideways over your head.

7. Land with your feet just inside your shoulder width.

8. After you land, pull your arms and legs back together.

9. Do the exercise as fast as you can, with as many repeats as you can in 20 seconds.

10. Adopt the standing position and do gentle jogging on the spot for 10 seconds.

11. Repeat the above.

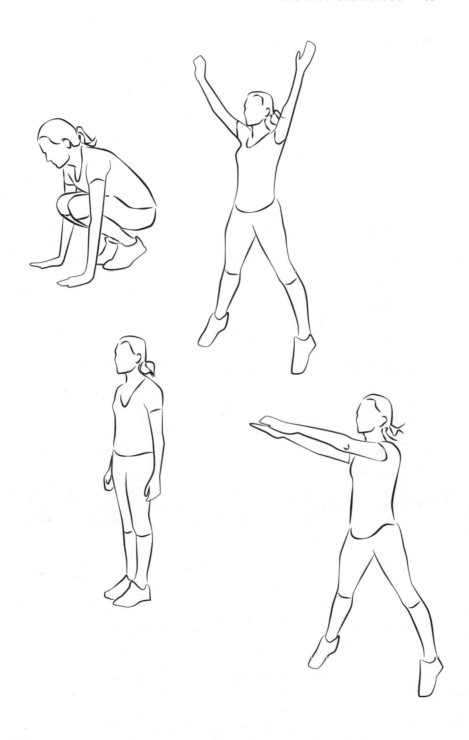

Toe-touch jacks (a variation on jumping jacks)

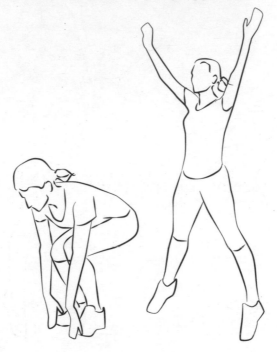

1. Stand with your knees slightly bent.

2. Squat down towards the ground.

3. Jump as high as you can, extending your arms and legs out to the side like a jumping jack.

4. Land with your feet just inside your shoulder width.

5. As you land, drop back into the squat position and touch your toes with your hands.

6. After you land, pull your arms and legs back together.

7. Do the exercise as fast as you can, with as many repeats as you can in 20 seconds.

8. Adopt the standing position and do gentle jogging on the spot for 10 seconds.

9. Repeat the above.

Ski moguls

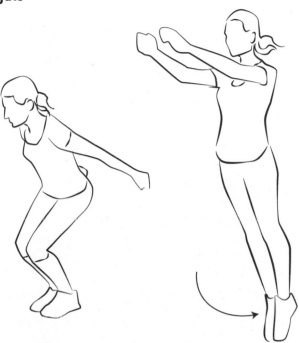

1. With your feet together, squat down and swing your arms behind you.

2. Jump up and to the right, swinging your arms in front of you, and landing in your start position.

3. Repeat the exercise as fast as you can, jumping from side to side.

4. Do this for 20 seconds.

5. Adopt the standing position and do gentle running on the spot for 10 seconds.

6. Repeat the above.

Advice Land as lightly as you can. Use your lower body and leg muscles to power your move and absorb the impact of your jump.

Mountain climbers

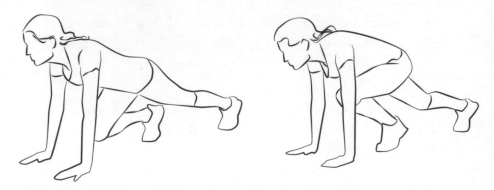

1. Place your hands on the floor, slightly further apart than shoulder width.

2. Place one foot forward with the leg bent under your body while the other foot is behind you with the leg extended back.

3. Keeping your upper body in place, alternate your foot and leg positions by pushing up your hips while immediately extending your forward leg back and pulling your rear leg forward under your body. Land on both feet simultaneously.

4. Do the exercise as fast as you can, with as many repeats as you can in 20 seconds.

5. Relax, move your arms around, gently move your legs for 10 seconds. Alternatively, stand up for 10 seconds and gently move your arms and feet. Take one or two deep breaths.

6. Repeat the above.

ADVICE Make sure your angle is perfect. The angle your legs move at is what will give you the desired results. Even if you work hard, if your angle is not correct, you will not get the desired results. The proper angle with your legs is vital and, equally important, you must keep correct posture. This is achieved by ensuring that your weight is distributed evenly between each of your feet and hands. During the exercise, your hips should be as low as possible and you should bring your knees as close to your chest as possible, ideally almost under your shoulders.

Sidewinder mountain climbers (a variation on mountain climbers)

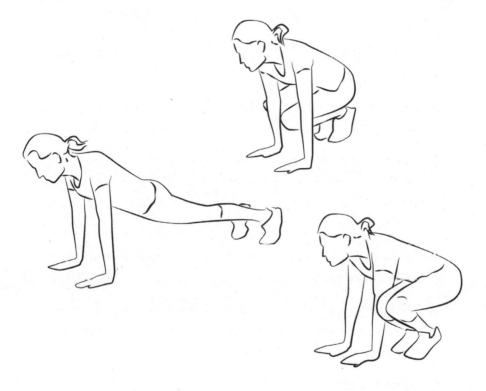

1. Place your hands on the floor, slightly further apart than shoulder width.

2. Place both feet behind you with your legs extended back.

3. Keeping your upper body in place, and, keeping your feet together all the time, jump your feet up forward under your body to land as close to your right hand as you can, then immediately jump your feet back again so that your legs are extended.

4. Then jump your feet forward under your body to land as close to your left hand as you can, then immediately jump your feet back again so your legs are extended.

5. Do the exercise as fast as you can, alternating your feet to each side, with as many repeats as you can in 20 seconds.

6. Relax, move your arms around, gently move your legs for 10 seconds. Alternatively, stand up for 10 seconds and gently move your arms and feet. Take one or two deep breaths.

7. Repeat the above.

ADVICE Make sure your angle is perfect. The angle your legs move at is what will give you the desired results. Even if you work hard, if your angle is not correct, you will not get the desired results. The proper angle with your legs is vital and, equally important, you must keep proper posture. This is achieved by ensuring that your weight is distributed evenly between each of your feet and hands. During the exercise your hips should be as low as possible.

Crunchy frogs

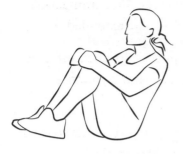 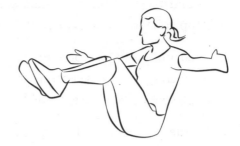

1. Sit on the floor and wrap your legs with your arms.

2. Quickly open yourself up by moving your arms out to your sides and extending your legs out in front of you.

3. Bring them back in.

4. Do as many repeats as you can in 20 seconds.

5. Relax for 10 seconds.

6. Repeat the above.

Scissor kicks

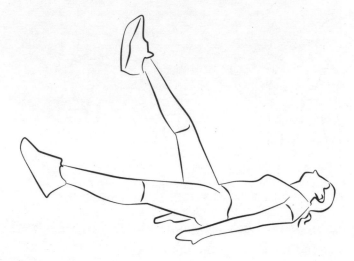

1. Lie on the floor.

2. Extend one leg up with the other raised in front. Keep both legs straight.

3. Do scissor-like motions with your legs while keeping your lower back pressed into the floor. If necessary, place your hands underneath your bottom.

4. Do as many repeats as you can in 20 seconds.

5. Relax for 10 seconds.

6. Repeat the above.

Push-ups

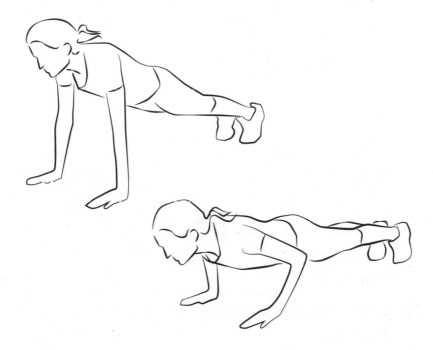

1. Get in a plank position with arms straight and hands a bit wider than shoulder width.

2. Lower your torso until your elbows form a 90-degree angle.

3. Push back up; keep your neck neutral.

4. Lower your torso again.

5. Do as many repeats as you can in 20 seconds.

6. Relax for 10 seconds.

7. Repeat the above.

Spiderman push-ups

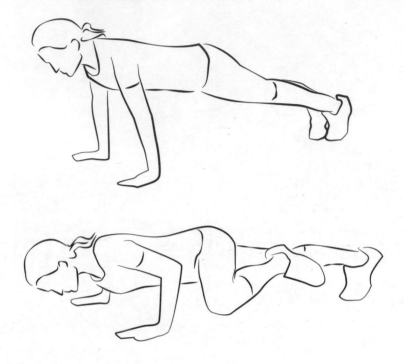

1. Start in a full plank position.

2. Perform a push-up and simultaneously draw one knee to the outside shoulder.

3. Return to plank and repeat while alternating sides.

4. Do as many repeats as you can in 20 seconds.

5. Relax for 10 seconds.

6. Repeat the above.

Kneeling diamond push-ups

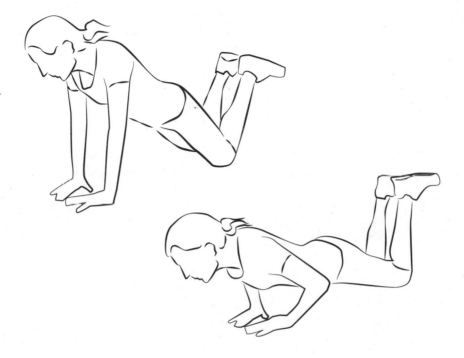

1. Get into a kneeling push-up position with your shoulders directly above your wrists.

2. Place your hands close together so that your thumbs and index fingers form a triangle on the floor.

3. Perform push-ups with your hands in this position.

4. Do as many repeats as you can in 20 seconds.

5. Relax for 10 seconds.

6. Repeat the above.

Plank hop-outs

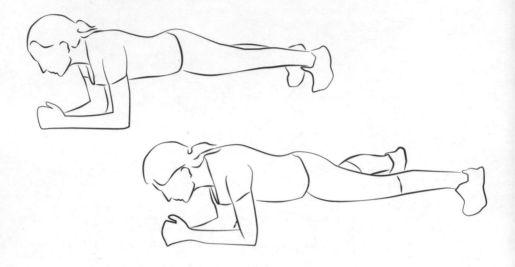

1. First, adopt the plank position by lying on your stomach with your feet together and toes tucked in and palms by your shoulders.

2. Lift your entire torso up off the ground, resting your forearms on the ground.

3. Now, start the hops: hop your feet out about 60cm (24in) away from each other and back in.

4. Do as many repeats of the hop as you can in 20 seconds.

5. Relax for 10 seconds.

6. Repeat the above.

Part Four

THE 12-MINUTE
WEIGHT-LOSS PLAN

Chapter Eight

SMART CARBS, UNSMART CARBS

THIS CHAPTER INTRODUCES YOU to the good and bad carbs — and this is essential knowledge for helping you to lose weight. Before we look at these, though, let's first ask whether dieting is the answer for rectifying weight gain.

DO WE HAVE TO DIET TO LOSE WEIGHT?

The short answer to the question of whether it is necessary to diet to lose weight is no. It is not only unnecessary to diet, but dieting is actually ineffective for most people. But before we go on, we need to be clear what we mean by dieting.

A little while ago I carried out a survey on 100 people. More than nine in every ten people defined dieting as eating much less food than usual or eating food that is significantly different from usual, or both. Again, around nine out of ten people agreed that what they regarded as dieting was unsustainable in the long term. Most regarded dieting as a short-term fix.

Almost nine out of ten people did not regard the minor changes that I describe in the next few chapters as dieting.

So what are these minor changes. Before we go into them over the next few chapters, let's have a look at the major nutrients in our diet and see how we might 'tweak' them to get the best out of them without actually 'going on a diet'.

FINDING THE TRUTH ABOUT CARBS

'All carbs are good'; 'All carbs are bad.' Which is right? Your answer will depend on whom you believe. If you are a fan of low-fat diets, such as Weight Watchers, you will believe that it is only fats in your diet that matter and that the carbohydrates – or 'carbs' – are completely unimportant. Watch your fat intake and the carbs will take care of themselves. But if you are a fan of high-protein/low-carbohydrate diets, such as the original Atkins (which I still find people wanting to follow) or the induction phase of the New Atkins Diet, the message you will have received loud and clear is that, provided you virtually eliminate all carbohydrates, the types of fats are unimportant. Eat as much artery-clogging fat as you like, you will still lose weight.

So where does the truth lie? The answer is with neither – time for a short lesson in nutrition and biology.

THE ENERGY PRODUCERS

Our bodies need three sources of fuel: fats, carbs and proteins. Carbs are the fuels the body prefers as a source of glucose energy. Protein is converted to glucose if carbs aren't available. What about fat? This is the emergency fuel that is stored in case we starve. When food enters the stomach, special chemicals called enzymes break it down so that the fats, carbs and proteins are absorbed into the bloodstream as small molecules. In the case of carbs these molecules are glucose.

Let's look at what happens to carbs, or glucose, next. They meet a hormone: insulin. The job of insulin, which is secreted by the pancreas gland, is to push glucose into our cells, where it is converted to energy or stored as a larger chemical called glycogen. But that is not all that insulin does. One of its other important actions is to store fat.

INSULIN CAN MAKE US FAT

When we eat carbs, the resultant glucose causes the release of insulin. The more glucose in our blood the more insulin we produce. And the more insulin we produce the more fat gets stored in our bodies – in other words, the fatter we get. And if we keep pushing insulin too much, eventually it can't do its job of converting glucose to energy properly so we have to produce more insulin to do the job. This is called glucose intolerance. Our cells become resistant to insulin, which is why we then need higher and higher levels of it. The result? High levels of insulin create more and more fat in our bodies, so we put on weight. Eventually, insulin resistance reaches a level when we become diabetic. That is what a particular kind of diabetes, known as type-2 diabetes, is: insulin resistance. Or, if it doesn't result in diabetes, it can cause a condition known as the metabolic syndrome (once called syndrome X). This is a group of clinical features that includes: high blood pressure; abdominal obesity (too much fat around the waist – the most dangerous place to store fat in terms of heart disease); glucose intolerance; and abnormal levels of blood fats (high triglycerides and low HDL or 'good' cholesterol).

Now, up to this point, fans of low-carb diets have got it right.

But from this point on they are completely wrong. You see, every carb is digested and absorbed at a different rate with different effects on blood levels of glucose; for example, white bread causes a rapid rise in blood glucose, whereas an apple causes a much lower rise. And, of course, the quicker the rise and the higher the level of blood glucose, the more insulin is produced. And the more rapid and higher the rise, the more rapid the subsequent *fall* in blood glucose.

THE CAUSES OF HUNGER POST-MEAL

Most of us have experienced the feeling of fullness immediately after eating a Chinese meal followed by hunger only two hours later. Why does this happen? Simply, the carbs in a Chinese meal, especially the white rice, cause rapid high levels of blood sugar, which satisfies hunger, followed by rapid falls, but this makes us feel hungry again.

Look at what happens when we eat a meal that starts off perhaps with a small portion of pasta cooked *al dente* (tender but with a bite in the centre), followed by a main course of your favourite meat or fish with new potatoes and lots of green vegetables, followed by fruit salad (and, go on, have some custard too, if you like!). The amount of carbs might be the same, perhaps even higher, than in the Chinese meal, but the resulting blood glucose levels are much lower. Why? Because these kinds of carbs are digested and absorbed much more slowly, so we feel satisfied and we don't feel ravenous again two hours later. Just as importantly, our insulin levels haven't been pushed sky high. It's the rapid rises that are the problem.

THE GLYCEMIC INDEX – A WAY TO MEASURE CARBS

All carbs, therefore, are different. Some cause rapid rises in blood glucose, whereas others cause only gentle rises. The rate at which a particular carb causes blood glucose to rise is called its glycemic index, or GI for short. A carb with a low GI causes gentle blood glucose rises, whereas a carb with a high GI causes steep rises. This means that low-GI carbs cause only gentle insulin production, whereas high-GI carbs cause high insulin production. Later in this chapter you will find a list of many common carbs divided into low, medium and high GI.

Incidentally, if you ever knew it, forget all that nonsense about 'complex carbohydrates', such as potatoes, being better for your blood glucose than 'simple carbohydrates', such as white flour. That was based on pseudo-science, which has been completely disproved. The chemical structure of a carb is no pointer to what it does to your blood glucose. The only way to find out, and the way researchers have discovered the GI values of carbs, is by laboriously feeding volunteers different carb foods and then measuring their blood glucose responses over a period of several hours. That is why the GI values are not yet available for every food, but we have enough information to work out a healthy and effective weight-loss diet.

Why is the GI value different for various carbs?

To answer that question we need to look at what exactly a carb is. The simplest carb is a monosaccharide ('mono' meaning one, 'saccharide' meaning sweet). The most common monosaccharide is glucose. If two monosaccharides are joined together, we have a disaccharide ('di' meaning two), the commonest example being sucrose or what we all know as table sugar. If lots of monosaccharides are joined together, we get polysaccharides ('poly' meaning many), and these are known as starches which, unlike monosaccharides and disaccharides, are not sweet. Two common starches are amylose and amylopectin, the importance of which we'll see in a moment.

Another group of carbohydrates made up of lots of different monosaccharides are dietary fibres. The main difference between fibres and other carbs, such as sugar and starches, is that they are not broken down by the body's digestive system, so they arrive at the large bowel unchanged.

Now, we can look at why different carbs have different GI values.

1. The less a starch swells up when it is cooked (the technical term for which is 'gelatinised'), the more slowly it is digested, and so the lower the GI. Examples of less starch gelatinisation, and so low GI, are long-grain rice, brown rice and *al dente* spaghetti. More gelatinisation, and so higher GI, is seen in sticky white rice and overcooked pasta.

2. The more fibrous a food is, the slower its digestion. This is because the fibrous coat around seeds and plant cells provides a physical barrier. Examples of fibrous food are wholemeal bread, pumpernickel bread, lentils, All-Bran and barley, all of which have a low GI. Low-fibre foods, with a high GI, include cornflakes and bagels.

3. The more amylose a food contains compared with amylopectin, the less the starch swells and the slower it is digested. Foods with a high amylose-to-amylopectin content, and therefore a low GI, include basmati rice, sweet potatoes and small new potatoes, whereas foods with a high amylopectin content and high GI include white rice and potatoes other than small new ones.

4. The less processed a food is, the larger the size of its particles and the more difficult it is for water and digestive enzymes to penetrate the higher surface area of the particles. This results in lower GI values, as seen in stoneground wholemeal bread and rolled oats. Highly processed foods with a high GI include instant oats, rice cakes and white bread.

5. Acidic foods slow down stomach emptying, which slows down the rate at which starch is digested. Good examples are sourdough bread and puddings made from sourdough.

6. Surprisingly, the digestion of sugar produces far fewer glucose molecules than does the digestion of starch. For this reason some breakfast cereals and some biscuits that are quite high in sugar actually have fairly low GI values, but, although they may have a low GI, it doesn't mean that eating a lot of them is healthy, as too much sugar is unhealthy.

7. Fat also slows down stomach emptying and so slows down the digestion of starch. This is the reason that potato crisps have a lower GI than boiled or baked potatoes. Not that that makes potato crisps healthy – after all, they still contain a lot of fat.

As we saw earlier, the GI values of food cannot be predicted. They have to be worked out by measuring blood glucose levels after each food has been eaten. This has to be done on a large number of volunteers and on different samples of the same food type, and this is the reason you will find variations in published GI values of foods. Also, the way a food is cooked will affect its GI value. As we have seen, overcooked pasta has a much higher GI than pasta that is cooked *al dente*.

First, here is a simple guide to the significance of a food's GI value:

GI less than 40:   very low GI

GI 40–55:   low GI

GI 55–70:   medium GI

GI more than 70:   high GI

Rice is food whose GI varies according to its variety. This is because different rices contain different amounts of the starch, amylose. Amylose is digested slowly, and the more that is present, the lower the GI. Here are some typical GI values:

THE GI VALUES OF RICES

Rices	Comments	GI value
Parboiled rice	During parboiling water-soluble nutrients pass from the outer layers to the inner, which makes this rice very nutritious	44
Uncle Ben's rice (which is parboiled)	As parboiled rice	44
Short-grain Japanese rice	This has a surprisingly low-GI value, which probably contributes to the low prevalence of coronary heart disease in Japan	48
Brown rice	Long- or medium-grain nutty-flavoured rice – the most nutritious rice	55
Long-grain white rice	Provided it isn't overcooked and the rice grains remain separate	56
Basmati rice	Its lower GI value is due to its high amylose content	58
Instant rice	Commercially pre-cooked in order to shorten preparation time in the home	87
Pudding rice	A high GI is due to the absence of amylose	88

Below is a table of GI values of some common foods. Don't treat the figures as gospel – there are enormous variations in samples of food depending on where it is grown or processed, how ripe it is (in the case of fruit), and how well cooked it is. Different researchers have found quite a variety of values for what would seem to be identical foods. This is why you may find different values for the same food in different books. As I have said earlier, working out the GI values of foods is not an exact science and there are all kinds of factors that can cause wide variations, so treat these figures as a rough guideline only.

GI VALUES OF SOME COMMON FOODS

Food	GI
BREADS AND BAKERY	
Bagel, white	72
Baguette, white, plain	95
Chapatti	58
Fruit loaf	44
Hamburger bun	61
Melba toast	70
Pumpernickel bread	50
Wholemeal rye bread	58
Rye bread	65
Sourdough rye	53
White-flour bread	70
Wholemeal wheat-flour bread	71
Wholemeal flour	52
Multigrain	49
100% wholemeal bread	51
Pitta bread, white	57
Muffins, blueberry	59

▶

Food	GI
BISCUITS	
Digestives	59
Oatcakes	57
Rich Tea	55
Shortbread	64
CRACKERS	
Cream crackers	65
Puffed rice cakes, white	78
Rye crispbread	64
Water biscuit	71
Wheat crackers	67
BREAKFAST CEREALS AND RELATED PRODUCTS	
All-Bran	42
Bran Flakes	74
Coco Pops	77
Cornflakes	81
Frosties	55
Muesli	49
Oat bran, raw	55
Porridge made from rolled oats	58
Porridge, instant	66
Puffed Wheat	74
Rice Krispies	82
Shredded Wheat	75
Special K	69
Sultana Bran	73
Weetabix	70
Couscous	65
Rice, white, boiled	64
Basmati, white, boiled	58
Brown rice	55
Glutinous rice	92
Instant rice, white, boiled	69

▶

Food	GI
Jasmine rice	109
Long-grain, boiled	48
Parboiled rice	60
Rice cracker, plain	91
Uncle Ben's (parboiled) rice	42
DAIRY PRODUCTS AND ALTERNATIVES	
Custard	38
Ice cream, regular	61
Ice cream, low-fat	43
Milk, full-fat	27
Milk, skimmed	32
Milk, condensed, sweetened	61
Yoghurt, natural	36
Yoghurt, fruit, low-fat	26
SOYA-BASED MILK	
Soya milk, full-fat	40
Soya milk, reduced-fat	44
FRUIT AND FRUIT PRODUCTS	
Apples, raw	38
Apple juice, unsweetened	40
Apricots, raw	57
Apricots, tinned	64
Apricots, dried	31
Banana, raw	52
Cherries, raw	22
Dates, dried	103
Figs, dried	61
Grapefruit, raw	25
Grapefruit juice, unsweetened	48
Grapes, raw	46
Kiwi fruit, raw	53
Lychee, tinned	79

▶

Food	GI
Mango, raw	51
Marmalade, orange	48
Oranges, raw	42
Orange juice	52
Papaya, raw	59
Peaches, raw	42
Peaches, tinned	38
Peach, tinned in natural juice	45
Pears, raw	38
Pears, tinned in natural juice	43
Pineapple, raw	59
Pineapple juice, unsweetened	46
Plums, raw	39
Prunes, pitted	29
Raisins	64
Strawberries, fresh	40
Strawberry jam	51
Sultanas	56
Tomato juice, unsweetened	38
Watermelon, raw	72
PULSES AND NUTS	
Baked beans, tinned	40
Beans, dried, boiled	29
Butter beans	31
Haricot beans	38
Hummus	6
Kidney beans	28
Lentils	26
Soya beans	18
MIXED MEALS AND CONVENIENCE FOODS	
Chicken nuggets	46
Fish fingers	38

▶

Food	GI
Pizza, cheese	60
Pizza, vegetarian, thin and crispy	49
Stuffed grapevine leaves (rice and lamb stuffing with tomato sauce)	30
White bread with butter	59
White bread with skimmed-milk cheese	55
White bread with butter and skimmed-milk cheese	62
White/wholemeal bread with peanut butter	59

PASTA, NOODLES AND GNOCCHI

Food	GI
Fettucine, egg	40
Gluten-free	54
Gnocchi	68
Instant noodles	48
Linguine, thick, durum wheat	46
Linguine, thin, durum wheat	52
Macaroni	47
Ravioli, durum wheat flour, meat-filled	39
Rice noodles, dried, boiled	61
Rice noodles, freshly made, boiled	40
Rice vermicelli	58
Spaghetti, white, boiled 5 min	38
Spaghetti, white, boiled 10 min	42
Spaghetti, white, boiled 20 min	61
Spaghetti, wholemeal, boiled	32
Vermicelli, white, boiled	35

SNACK FOODS AND CONFECTIONERY

Food	GI
Chocolate, milk, plain	43
Corn chips	63
Jelly beans	78
Mars bar	65
Muesli bar containing dried fruit	61
Cashew nuts, salted	22
Peanuts	14

▶

Food	GI
Popcorn, plain	72
Potato crisps, plain, salted	54
Honey	55
VEGETABLES	
Peas	48
Sweetcorn	54
Beetroot	64
Carrots	47
Parsnips	97
Potato, baked	85
Potato, boiled	50
Potato, French fries	75
Potato, instant mashed	85
Potato, mashed	74
Potato, new	57
Sweet potato	61
Swede	72
Yam	37
BEVERAGES	
Cola drink	63
Lucozade	58
Juices	95
Apple juice	40
Grapefruit juice, unsweetened	40
Orange juice	48
Pineapple juice, unsweetened	50
Tomato juice, canned, no added sugar	46

THE GLYCEMIC LOAD: COMBINING THE QUALITY WITH PORTION SIZE OF CARBS

You may have heard about the GL (glycemic load) of a food and might be confused about the difference between GI and GL. A question I'm sometimes asked is, which is more useful to know: the glycemic index (GI) or glycemic load (GL)? To answer that, let's first look at the difference between them.

Both the quality and the quantity of carbs impact our glycemic response to a food or meal. The GI gives us a measure of carb *quality* by comparing equal quantities of available carbs in foods as we have seen in the lists above. By contrast, the GL is the *product* of a food's GI and its total available carb content, so the GL gives us the relative glycemic impact *of a typical serving* of a particular food.

On the face of it, you might think that GL is more useful than GI, but research (published by Hodge, et al., 'Glycemic index and dietary fiber and the risk of type 2 diabetes', *Diabetes Care*, November 2004) contrasted the potential benefits of moderately high-carbohydrate diets with a low GI versus diets that have a lower GL by virtue of a low carb content, in other words a lower quantity of carbs overall.

In their analysis of 36,000 adults followed for four years, the researchers found that higher-carbohydrate diets were associated with a lower risk of development of type-2 diabetes; however, the *type* of carb was equally important: low-GI carbs reduced the risk, whereas high-GI carbs increased the risk. So low GI and low GL are not equivalent and produce different clinical outcomes. This would apply not only to diabetes but also to weight control. The essential point of the paper is that focusing on GI is more important than focusing on GL.

The simplest way to consume a moderately high-carb but

low-GI diet is to incorporate the recommendations of the World Health Organization/Food and Agriculture Organization:

> The glycemic index can be used, in conjunction with information about food composition, to guide food choices. For practical application, the glycemic index is useful to rank foods by developing exchange lists of categories of low glycemic index foods, such as legumes [pulses], pearled barley, lightly refined grains (e.g. whole grain pumpernickel bread, or breads made from coarse flour), pasta, etc. Specific local foods should be included in such lists where information is available (e.g. green bananas in the Caribbean and specific rice varieties in Southeast Asia).
>
> In choosing carbohydrate foods, both glycemic index and food composition must be considered. Some low GI foods may not always be a good choice because they are high in fat. Conversely, some high GI foods may be a good choice because of convenience or because they have low energy and high nutrient content. It is not necessary or desirable to exclude or avoid all high GI foods.

In other words, GI should be used to compare foods of similar composition within food groups. By choosing the lower-GI options within a food category (breads, breakfast cereals, etc.), an individual automatically chooses those with a lower GL. Because most fruit and vegetables, other than potatoes, are not major contributors to carb intake, their GI should not be the basis for restriction.

The key message is that the evidence, as it stands, suggests that for preventing type-2 diabetes – and also for helping weight control – we ought to concentrate on low GI rather than on low GL.

Below is a table showing typical GI and GL values for usual portion sizes of some common foods and beverages:

TYPICAL GI AND GL VALUES OF COMMON FOODS AND DRINKS

(Note: The foods mentioned are present for information purposes and not necessarily because they are desirable.)

Food	GI	g/ml	GL
BAKERY PRODUCTS AND BREADS			
Bagel, white	72	70	25
Baguette, white	95	30	15
Barley bread	34	30	7
Beefburger bun	61	30	9
Hummus	6	30	0
Pitta bread, white	57	30	10
Pumpernickel bread	50	30	7
Sponge cake, plain	46	63	17
WhIte bread	70	30	10
Wholegrain bread	51	30	7
Wholemeal bread	71	30	9
BREAKFAST CEREALS AND RELATED PRODUCTS			
All-Bran	42	30	12
Coco Pops	77	30	20
Cornflakes	81	30	23
Grapenuts	75	30	16
Muesli	49	30	16
Oats (rolled oats)	55	250	13
Instant oats	83	250	30
Puffed wheat	74	30	17
Raisin Bran (Kellogg's)	61	30	12
Special K (Kellogg's)	69	30	14
GRAINS			
Brown rice	55	150	16
Bulgur wheat	48	150	12
Corn on the cob	53	150	20
Couscous	65	150	9

▶

Food	GI	g/ml	GL
Pearl barley	28	150	12
Quinoa	53	150	13
White rice (Uncle Ben's)	42	150	14
White rice, short-grain	69	150	43
BISCUITS AND CRACKERS			
Rice cakes	82	25	17
Rye crisps	64	25	11
Shortbread	64	25	10
Water biscuits	71	25	12
PASTA AND NOODLES			
Fettuccini, egg	40	180	15
Macaroni	47	180	23
Macaroni cheese	64	180	32
Spaghetti, white, *al dente*	38	180	22
Spaghetti, white, boiled until soft	61	180	26
Spaghetti, wholemeal, *al dente*	32	180	17
BEANS AND NUTS			
Baked beans	40	150	6
Cashew nuts, salted	27	50	3
Chickpeas, cooked	10	150	3
Chickpeas, tinned in brine	38	150	9
Kidney beans, cooked	28	150	7
Lentils, cooked	26	150	5
Peanuts	7	50	0
Soya beans, cooked	18	150	1
VEGETABLES			
Baked potato	85	150	33
Boiled potato	50	150	21
Carrots	47	80	2
Mashed potato, instant	87	150	17
Peas	48	80	4

▶

Food	GI	g/ml	GL
Sweet potato	61	150	22
Yam	37	150	20
FRUIT			
Apple	38	120	6
Banana	52	120	16
Grapefruit	25	120	3
Grapes	46	120	11
Orange	42	120	4
Peach	42	120	5
Peach, tinned in natural juice	45	120	5
Pear	38	120	4
Prunes	29	60	10
Raisins	64	60	28
Watermelon	72	120	4
DAIRY AND RELATED PRODUCTS			
Ice cream	61	50	6
Milk, full-fat	27	250	5
Milk, skimmed	32	250	4
Yoghurt, low-fat with fruit	26	200	11
SNACKS, NIBBLES AND CONVENIENCE FOODS			
Chicken nuggets	46	100	7
Corn chips	63	50	11
Microwave popcorn, plain	72	20	6
Potato crisps, plain	54	50	12
Pretzels	83	30	16
Snickers bar	51	60	18
BEVERAGES			
Apple juice, unsweetened	40	250	30
Cola drink	63	250	16
Orange juice, unsweetened	48	250	12
Tomato juice, tinned	46	250	4

You will also find more GI values in Chapter 24.

ALCOHOL

It's easy to forget about the carb content of alcoholic drinks, although for most drinks this is very small. Here are some typical drinks with their alcohol units, calorie and carb contents. Remember, all the carbs are sugars.

THE CALORIE AND CARB CONTENTS OF ALCOHOLIC DRINKS

	Alcohol units	Calories	Carb quantity
Red wine (125ml)	1.5–2	70	0.2g
Dry white wine (125ml)	1.5	65	0.6g
Medium white wine (125ml)	1.5	75	3g
Sweet white wine (125ml)	1.8	120	10g
Sherry (50ml)	1	135	6.9g
Port (50ml)	1	160	12g
Spirits (25ml)	1	220	trace
Cider (284ml)	1.5–2	30–60	2.6–5g

The question arises as to whether or not it's advisable to cut out alcohol on the 12-Minute Weight-Loss Plan. To answer, the impact of a small amount of alcohol, for example one glass a day or two to three times a week, has only a fairly modest impact. Anything more than that is something you should try to avoid, especially if you are in the losing-weight phase rather than the maintenance phase, having reached your target weight.

WHICH OTHER TYPES OF DRINKS ARE BEST AVOIDED?

Should we be avoiding other types of drinks, for general health reasons and to encourage weight loss? The following are the most potentially problematic.

Coffee

There is currently a strong debate about the good and the bad in coffee, especially its caffeine content. Barely a week goes by when the papers don't highlight some contradictory advice on the subject from so-called experts. There are so many aspects that it would be impossible to cover the subject, but it's worth mentioning two or three.

First, some sports enthusiasts find that drinking caffeinated coffee shortly before exercising gives them more energy and they are therefore able to benefit more from the exercise.

Second, caffeine in the evening may adversely affect your sleep, and there is evidence that poor sleep can lead to your metabolism not functioning properly, which, in turn, may make it more difficult for you to lose weight.

Third, what you put in your coffee is important. Sugar and full or semi-skimmed milk gives you unnecessary calories. Black coffee or coffee with a small amount of skimmed milk and no sugar is best for weight control.

Fruit juices

In recent years the media have quite rightly highlighted the high sugar content of fruit juices. Previously believed to be a healthy alternative, fruit juice has been known for a long time to damage the enamel of the teeth, but now it is being more frequently recognised that juices aren't kind to your waistline either.

A 150ml (5fl oz/¼ pint) serving of freshly squeezed orange juice, which is only a small glass, contains 64 kcal and 13.95g (½oz) sugar. Smooth orange juice made from concentrate contains 68 kcal and 15g (just over ½oz) sugar. I recommend avoiding fruit juices except as an occasional treat.

Smoothies

Although fruit smoothies might seem like a healthy way to consume fruits, they typically contain a fair amount of sugar. This is because the basic ingredients – fruit – contain sugar, which means that heavy fruit smoothies often have more sugar than a cola drink. A smoothie usually contains several pieces of fruit, which is a lot more than the one serving we would normally eat as whole fruit. A 250ml (9fl oz) serving of a smoothie containing white grape juice, peach purée, raspberry purée, apple and aronia juice might typically contain 135 kcal and 31.25g (over 1oz) sugars. Another smoothie containing purées of raspberry, banana and cranberry with apple and red grape juice might typically contain 108 kcal and 23g (just under 1oz) sugars.

Smoothies contain beneficial antioxidants from the fruit (or vegetables) but, nevertheless, fruit smoothies should be drunk fairly infrequently – perhaps once or twice a week. Vegetable smoothies, however, are much healthier and can be drunk much more often, such as daily.

SEASONAL CRAVINGS

Do you find that winter brings on food cravings? Many of us find that the cold weather and shorter days make us think more about food, especially high-carb foods such as potatoes, bread and biscuits. Why is this?

To understand what is happening at this time of the year, let's first look at what happens during summer. We have higher levels of vitamin D during the summer, because of the sun, and these higher levels boost the production of serotonin – otherwise known as the 'happy hormone'. In winter, there's less sun, so we have less vitamin D and less serotonin. So what do we do? We look for foods that boost our serotonin levels. And you can guess which foods do that the best – of course, it's carbs.

How do carbs exert this magical effect? First, they contain a lot of an amino acid called tryptophan, and this converts into serotonin. Second, carbs boost insulin levels in our body, and insulin allows tryptophan to cross the blood-brain barrier. Once in the brain, tryptophan converts to serotonin. So next time you have a mince pie at Christmas, remember all you're doing is boosting your levels of brain serotonin!

Does it matter if we boost our serotonin levels? Of course not, but ask the question, does it matter how food cravings boost serotonin, and the answer is yes, it does. And the reason is that an intake of food high in refined carbs produces rapid rises in our insulin levels, and insulin has one unfortunate effect: it causes us to put down more fat in our body's fat cells. Which means we put on weight. Not only that, if we repeatedly give in to our carb cravings, our bodies get so used to insulin that we have to produce

▶

more and more – a condition known as *insulin resistance*, which eventually leads to type-2 diabetes.

What, then, can we do about winter carb cravings? One solution is to eat protein with or just before carbs. This will reduce the rapid blood sugar highs. If you really can't resist a sweet or chocolate, therefore, try to have it only after a meal that has contained protein. And the next time you can't resist a mince pie, eat it with low-fat or fat-free yoghurt sweetened with artificial sweetener (see page 143) and, for a little Christmas magic, a dash of brandy. It will be much healthier than brandy custard or cream – and still taste delicious! Who said you can't lose weight without foregoing your favourite foods?

Finally, if you find you have an irresistible craving for a high-carb food, try some of these tips:

▶ Distract yourself – boredom often brings on cravings, so throwing yourself into some mental or physical activity will often help the craving to pass.

▶ Close your eyes for a few moments and imagine the particular craved food crawling with flies – you might find you can resist it now!

▶ If you really must give in, take one or two chocolates or sweets – or whatever the food is – from their container, put the container back, and then eat the food very slowly, savouring each mouthful. Enjoy the food for its quality, not its quantity.

Carbs are not the whole story for people who want to lose weight, of course. Another vitally important factor is the second major nutrient in our diets: fats. More about those later.

Chapter Nine

CAN YOU EAT A RAINBOW?

B EFORE WE LEAVE CARBS ENTIRELY, let's take a closer look at the largest carb group: fruit and vegetables. After all, the inclusion of fruit and veg is essential for a normal, healthy diet.

Let me start by asking you, can you eat a rainbow? If you think the answer is no, let me show you why you might want to rethink your answer, and why it's important to try to eat a rainbow every day.

Twenty years ago doctors began to realise that fruit and vegetables can help to prevent cancers. This is because of the foods' chemicals, known as phytochemicals. In particular, fruits and vegetables with the most vibrant colours seemed to be the most beneficial. One of the best examples is beta-carotene, which gives carrots their bright orange colour. With time, doctors discovered what were the different pigments contained in each of the foods. They also realised that the health benefits went far beyond cancers: they included the prevention of many other diseases, especially coronary heart disease.

Let's take a look at the health-giving properties of some fruit and vegetables – the rainbow of colours.

RED/PINK

Foods that are red or pink in colour contain lycopenes, which help to prevent some cancers, especially of the prostate, and phenols, which may help to reduce the risk of cancer, heart disease and infections.

Beetroot	Red cabbage
Guavas	Red pepper
Pink grapefruit	Tomato
Radish	Watermelon

ORANGE

Beta-carotene is present in orange-coloured fruit and veg. It is perhaps the most well-known antioxidant and it protects the body's cells from a wide range of diseases, as well as being good for eye and skin health.

Apricot	Mango
Cantaloupe melon	Pumpkin, acorn and butternut squash
Carrot	Sweet potato

ORANGE/YELLOW

Foods that are orange/yellow, contain beta-cryptoxanthin, another antioxidant that prevents cell damage.

Lemon	Peach
Nectarine	Pineapple
Orange	Tangerine
Papaya	Yellow grapefruit

YELLOW/GREEN

Fruit and vegetables that are yellow/green in colour contain lutein and zeaxanthin, which are good for the eyes by helping to prevent cataracts and macular degeneration – both common causes of blindness.

Avocado	Green bean
Cos and Romaine lettuce	Honeydew melon
Courgette	Kiwi fruit
Cucumber	Mustard and cress
Green and yellow peppers	Spinach

GREEN

Vegetables and fruit that are green contain sulforaphane, isothiocyanates and indoles, which help the liver flush out toxins.

Beans	Cauliflower	Spinach
Broccoli	Globe artichokes	Turnip
Brussels sprouts	Kale	
Cabbage	Peas	

GREEN/WHITE

The green/white group contains flavonoids, which stimulate the production of glutathione, which in turn helps to prevent cancer. The alliums (onions and leeks) contain organosulfur compounds, which also help to protect against cancer.

Asparagus	Garlic
Cannellini bean	Leeks
Celery	Mushrooms
Chive	Onion
Endive	Shallot

BLUE/PURPLE/DARK RED

Fruit and veg with these colours contain anthocyanins, which prevent blood clots and therefore help to reduce the risk of coronary heart disease.

Aubergine	Raspberry
Beetroot	Red apple skin
Blackberry, blackcurrant, blueberry, bilberry	Red grape, red grape juice, red wine
Cherry	Red pepper
Plum	Strawberry
Prune	

When you plan the food for your day, include plenty of fresh vegetables and some fruit, and aim to eat a rainbow every day.

Chapter Ten

SMART FATS, UNSMART FATS

ALL FATS ARE BAD. RIGHT? Of course, that's wrong but, as with carbs, it's a question of quantity and quality – how much and what kind.

We need some dietary fat for our health. Fats supply essential fatty acids and are important for making available to our bodies the fat-soluble vitamins A, D, E and K and for building body tissue. There are two main kinds of fats and oils, and all fatty foods contain them in different proportions. They are:

SATURATED FATS

These fats are solid at room temperature, and, despite some recent research to the contrary, many doctors believe they clog up arteries. Examples of foods containing large quantities of saturated fats are fatty meats, poultry skin and full-fat dairy products, such as whole milk and cream. Palm and coconut oils are also high in saturated fats.

UNSATURATED FATS

These are oils, which means they are liquid at room temperature. Some oils contain mostly polyunsaturates, which are liquid even at fridge temperatures. Examples are corn oil, safflower oil, soya oil and sunflower oil. One particularly beneficial type of polyunsaturate is omega-3 fatty acids, found in oily fish (such as fresh or smoked salmon, mackerel, sardines, herring and white albacore tuna), flaxseed and omega-3-fortified eggs. We'll look at omega-3s in more detail in the next chapter. Other unsaturated oils are monounsaturates. These are thick but not completely hard at fridge temperatures. They are the healthiest, and are found in nuts (especially almonds, cashew nuts, pistachio nuts, peanuts and peanut butter), olives and olive oil, rapeseed oil and avocados.

THE EFFECTS OF DIFFERENT FATS ON THE BODY

The main concern is the effect of the different kinds of fats and oils on our blood fats and our hearts, explained below.

There are two important ones – cholesterol and triglycerides (a blood fat). With regard to cholesterol, there are two main types: LDL (which stands for low-density lipoprotein), which is the naughty stuff that clogs up our arteries; and HDL (high-density lipoprotein), which is the good type that protects our arteries. Levels of both are affected by diet. HDL is also affected by exercise (which increases it) and smoking (which lowers it).

Triglycerides are also important for lots of health reasons, but especially for our hearts. Too many of them and our risk of coronary heart disease rises.

Saturated fats increase LDL (bad cholesterol) and too many of them are bad for the heart. Polyunsaturates lower LDL, although they unfortunately also lower HDL (good cholesterol). Used in small amounts occasionally, however, they are useful for cooking at high temperatures. Monounsaturates are the best. They both lower LDL and raise HDL, and are very healthy for the heart. Diets high in saturated fats and trans-fats are closely linked with insulin resistance.

A word about most margarines: these are vegetable oils that used to be artificially saturated (hydrogenated) to make them semi-solid. Nowadays, a process called intereserification is used with the purpose of making the margarine safer; however, many experts are still concerned that this new type of chemically constructed fat is not good for us, especially those of us with diabetes, heart disease or weight problems.

You can see that the best fats to include in your diet, whether or not you are trying to lose weight, are those with lots of monounsaturates and polyunsaturates (especially omega-3 oils), so what are the best ways to achieve this?

▶ Avoid fatty meats and poultry skin.

▶ Eat oily fish. If you don't like fish, consider taking omega-3 fish oil supplements.

▶ Drink skimmed, or at the very least semi-skimmed, milk and eat low-fat cheeses such as cottage cheese, feta and ricotta.*

▶ Choose light margarine or margarine that is labelled polyunsaturated and trans-fat-free. Use light margarine instead of butter or ordinary margarine, or use butter in *very* sparing amounts.

▶ Use low-fat or fat-free mayonnaise and salad dressings.*

▶ Buy foods that are labelled low-fat.*

▶ Cook with liquid oils rather than solid fats. Especially good are olive, rapeseed and sesame oils.

► Bake or steam rather than sauté or fry.

► Eat fewer commercially prepared baked goods, snack foods and processed foods, including fast foods.

► Try to avoid foods containing hydrogenated or partially hydrogenated oils. Or at least choose food products that list the hydrogenated oils near to the end of the ingredient list (which means the amount present is likely to be very small).

* See below about low-fat food choices.

The central message of my book is that it is not necessary – indeed, for most people, it is *undesirable* – to diet. But this doesn't mean we shouldn't make healthy food choices. And one of those food choices is to focus on good fats (monounsaturates and polyunsaturates) while steering away from bad fats (saturated fats and trans-fats). The good fats help sugar and insulin metabolism, which helps long-term weight loss, while the bad fats damage sugar and insulin metabolism, which makes weight gain very likely after initial weight loss.

All of us need healthy diets regardless of whether or not we want to lose weight. A healthy diet has a good balance of proteins, fats and carbs. In the last chapter we saw how to choose the good carbs. In this chapter we have seen how to choose the good fats, so there is absolutely no need to avoid carbs and equally there is no need to avoid fats. Instead, choose smart carbs and smart fats. This way you can still enjoy eating a diet full of flavoursome food without having to 'go on a diet'.

THE PROBLEM WITH LOW-FAT FOODS

Over the past two or three decades the media have, quite rightly, reported on the importance of cutting back on our intake of fats, especially saturated fats. Food manufacturers have taken this on board. Unfortunately, low-fat food can be less palatable, so food manufacturers have had to find ways of dealing with this challenge.

One way is to replace saturated fats with unsaturated vegetable oils, which have been hydrogenated to make them solid or semi-solid. The downside is that hydrogenated fats increase levels of dangerous trans-fats – these are bad both for our cholesterol and the heart and have been linked to cancer. The media have rightly highlighted this issue, which has forced food manufacturers to find yet other ways to improve the taste and texture of our food. One way is to increase the amount of sugar in food products. And the result? Many low-fat products are high in carbs. These foods, while low in fat, can result in blood sugar swings, because of their high refined-carb content with the resultant increased risk of obesity, diabetes and heart disease. In other words, some low-fat foods can be just as unhealthy as high-fat ones!

So what's the answer? Because not all low-fat foods are high in carbs, it's important to read the nutrition labels.

Below is a nutrition label from the back of a loaf of white bread.

Nutrition

Typical values	100g contains	Each slice (typically 44g) contains	% RI*	RI* for an average adult
Energy	985kJ	435kJ		8400kJ
	235kcal	105kcal	5%	2000kcal
Fat	1.5g	0.7g	1%	70g
of which saturates	0.3g	0.1g	1%	20g
Carbohydrate	45.5g	20.0g		
of which sugars	3.8g	1.7g	2%	90g
Fibre	2.8g	1.2g		
Protein	7.7g	3.4g		
Salt	1.0g	0.4g	7%	6g

This pack contains 16 servings
*Reference intake of an average
adult (8400kJ / 2000kcal)

The nutrition information

Typically, a nutrition label shows the nutritional content of 100g (3½oz) and a typical portion size, in this case one slice of bread. The label also indicates the proportion of the daily reference (that is, recommended) intake (RI) for adults for each nutrient. The label is likely to show:

▶ energy, expressed both as kj (kilojoules) and kcal (kilocalories = what most of us refer to as 'calories')

▶ fat, expressed as g (grams)

▶ saturated fats, in g

▶ carbs, in g

▶ of which sugars, in g

▶ protein, in g

▶ fibre, in g

▶ salt, in g

The label tells us whether or not the amount of each nutrient is too high or too low according to current guidelines. Our concerns are with fat, saturated fat, sugar and salt, so it's useful to make a note of the guidelines for 100g (3½oz) of each of these nutrients:

Total fat	3–17.5g
Saturated fat	1.5–5g
Sugars	5–12.5g
Salt	0.3–1.5g = 0.1 to 0.6g sodium

So an ideal low-fat, low-sugar food contains for each 100g (3½oz) no more than:

17.5g of total fat
5g of saturated fat
12.5g of sugars

(The above sugar amount of 12.5g is actually equivalent to 3¼ tsp sugar. It's best to try to wean yourself off sugar and have it only as a treat occasionally.)

Similar information is often displayed on the front of pre-packed food. But there is one major difference. The nutritional information is usually for a typical portion size, which of course begs the question of what is a typical portion size? There is often quite a lot of other nutritional information on pre-packed foods. One useful type is colour coding – called the traffic-light system – which can be helpful for quickly spotting if a food is high, medium or low in fat, saturated fat, sugars and salt.

red = high
amber = medium
green = low

The more foods you eat with the green 'light', the better. Reds should be reserved for occasional consumption.

Keeping track of sugar

Added sugars shouldn't make up more than 10 per cent of our daily calorie intake from food and drink. This will vary depending on a person's size, age and level of physical activity. As a rough guide, daily added sugars shouldn't amount to more than 70g (2½oz) for men and 50g (1¾oz) for women.

With regard to sugars, my advice is to look for the 'carbohydrates (of which sugars)' figure on the nutrition label. This will show the sugar content for every 100g (3½oz). More than 12.5g (less than ½oz) of total sugars is high; less than 5g (⅛oz) is low. The Food Standards Agency (FSA) traffic-light signpost labelling system, explained above, gives the following colour code for sugars in **food**:

▶ **Green** if total sugars are equal to, or less than, 5g per 100g (3½oz).

▶ **Amber** if total sugars are more than 5g per 100g (3½oz) but less than, or equal to, 12.5g per 100g (3½oz).

▶ **Red** if total sugars are more than 12.5g per 100g (3½oz).

The FSA does not provide a traffic-light system for **drinks**, but it says that the criteria below should be followed if drinks manufacturers choose to apply traffic-light labelling to their products:

▶ **Green** if total sugars are equal to, or less than, 2.5g per 100ml (3½fl oz).

▶ **Amber** if total sugars are more than 2.5g per 100ml (3½fl oz) but less than, or equal to, 6.3g per 100ml (3½fl oz).

▶ **Red** if total sugars are more than 6.3g per 100ml (3½fl oz).

As you can see, the amount for drinks is *half* that for food.

The ingredients list

Most pre-packed foods show the ingredients in order of weight. In other words, the main ingredients come first. From this you can tell if the food is high in fat or sugar, or both. Because so many low-fat foods today are high in sugars, it's useful to be able to tell quickly if a particular food is high in sugars. A good rule of thumb is that if sugars are first or second in the list, then that food is high in sugars. Next time you're in a supermarket, look at the ingredients lists of, say, breakfast cereals. You may be surprised to see how many list sugars in their first two ingredients.

Chapter Eleven

ESSENTIAL OMEGA-3 AND OMEGA-6 FATS

B EFORE WE LEAVE THE SUBJECT of fats, let's look at essential fatty acids and especially omega-3 oils.

Essential fatty acids, or EFAs, are so called because our bodies cannot produce them, so we need them in our diet. They are important for several reasons, one being that they are used in the manufacture of substances called prostaglandins, which are essential for hundreds of bodily functions.

There are two types of EFA:

1. Omega-6 oils, such as linoleic acid, which we get from seed oils such as corn oil and sunflower.

2. Omega-3 oils, which we get from green leafy vegetables such as broccoli, spinach and lettuce; and fish oils such as those we get from oily fish such as mackerel, herring and salmon, and grass-fed lamb and beef.

Incidentally, omega-3 oils are particularly important in early life, so pregnant mums should make sure they have a good intake of these.

Certain conditions may interfere with the conversion of these oils to prostaglandins – fatty compounds that have important functions in our bodies. These conditions are: a diet rich in animal (or saturated) fats; too much alcohol; conditions such as diabetes and virus infections; and getting older. This is why EFA supplements are proving so popular.

EFAs are extremely important for our general health and, for example, for the prevention of heart disease. A good intake of EFAs will ensure a good level of prostaglandins, which will maximise the efficiency of the body's various metabolic processes.

OMEGA-3 FATS

The most interesting and most important fats of the two are the omega-3s, so let's take a closer look at them. There are three types:

1. Alpha-linolenic acid, found in green leafy vegetables, walnuts and pine nut oil, nuts and soya.

2. Docosahexaenoic acid (DHA), which comes from oily fish, especially mackerel, sardines, salmon and albacore tuna.

3. Eicosapentaenoic acid (EPA), which also comes from oily fish.

DHA and EPA, the omega-3s from fish, are the most powerful. They are especially important in the prevention and treatment of coronary heart disease, hypertension (high blood pressure), cancer and rheumatoid arthritis.

There are several ways that omega-3s help in heart disease:

▶ They increase levels of HDL (high-density lipoprotein) cholesterol. This is the 'good' cholesterol, which protects us from coronary heart disease. Remember, there are essentially two different kinds of cholesterol – HDL and LDL. LDL (low-density lipoprotein) cholesterol is the bad guy that clogs up our arteries, so we want as little LDL as possible and as much HDL as we can. The three main factors that affect cholesterol levels are: (1) smoking; (2) lack of exercise; and (3) a poor diet. All three push up LDL and lower HDL – bad news. So anything that lowers LDL and raises HDL is good. Cutting back on animal fats such as fatty meats and dairy products helps, as does having a lot of omega-3s.

▶ Omega-3s, especially from fish, push up HDL. These fats lower blood levels of triglycerides – another fat that is a risk factor for coronary heart disease. They reduce our risk of developing abnormal heart rhythms, which can cause sudden death. They also help to reduce high blood pressure, but only if taken in high quantities through supplements.

▶ They also reduce blood clotting, which in turn reduces the risk of clotting inside coronary arteries. This clotting is one important factor in causing heart attacks.

OMEGA-6 FATS

As we saw in Chapter 3 (What Makes Us Become Fat?) most people's diets are too high in omega-6 fats (which promotes inflammation) compared with omega-3s (which are anti-inflammatory), and this has a negative effect on our efforts to control our weight. Too many omega-6 fats increase the risk of many diseases, including heart disease, cancer and inflammatory and autoimmune disease (disease arising from an abnormal immune response of the body against substances and tissues normally present in the body, examples being many skin conditions and rheumatoid arthritis). By contrast, an increase in omega-3s is associated with a 70 per cent decrease in mortality in people with heart disease. Other known benefits of a lower omega-6 to omega-3 ratio include a decreased risk of breast cancer, less inflammation in rheumatoid arthritis, better asthma control and the reduced risk of spread from bowel cancer. Unfortunately, there is no single ideal omega-6 to omega-3 ratio, as the benefits vary from disease to disease.

How, therefore, can we try to correct the balance?

▶ Avoid vegetable oils high in omega-6. The worst are sunflower, corn, soya and cottonseed oils. The easiest way to reduce omega-6 is to cut out from the diet processed vegetable oils and processed foods that contain them. Margarine is a processed oil but is fine to use in very small amounts.

▶ Eat animal foods high in omega-3. We can do this by eating only lean cuts of meat and poultry and eating seafood, such as a fatty fish like salmon, once or twice a week. If you're not keen on fish, then consider taking supplements of omega-3.

SOME MYTHS ABOUT FATS

There is a lot of confusion about fatty foods – what's good and what's bad. Let's look at a few of the myths.

Vegetable oils

A popular myth is that all vegetable oils are good for you. But coconut oil and palm oil are both high in saturated fats, which are the fats that cause high cholesterol. Avoid these and opt instead for oils that are low in saturated fats. Good choices are nut oils, especially peanut, which contain mainly monounsaturated fats and are best for the heart.

Experiment with different oils

The qualities and flavours of different oils make them suitable for a variety of uses:

► As an all-purpose cooking and baking oil, use rapeseed or sesame or olive oil. Note that toasted sesame oil – the deep-brown variety – is best used sprinkled over stir-fry dishes at the end of cooking so as not to destroy its nutty flavour and aroma. The untoasted kind can be used for general frying, but care is needed, as it has a low burning point so should be cooked over a medium heat only.

► Try a nutty oil, such as walnut oil, for a salad dressing or baking. It contains a lot of omega-3 fat; however, it can go rancid quickly, so keep it in the fridge after opening.

► Use olive oil for Mediterranean food and salads. It's full of healthy monounsaturates and it adds a delicious flavour to foods, especially if you use extra-virgin varieties.

► For frying and roasting, use light olive oil or rapeseed oil.

► For stir-fries, try oils with a distinctive flavour. A little dash of toasted sesame oil can be added at the end of cooking.

► Non-stick vegetable oil cooking sprays are a good way of providing an almost negligible amount of fat when you need to prevent food from sticking to a pan.

CHEESE

When I worked as a physician in a well-known wellness clinic in London, I often found myself advising patients about their cholesterol levels. The common reply was, 'But I don't eat anything to cause high cholesterol.' A little digging found that, yes, their diet was very healthy except for one thing – they nearly all ate a lot of cheese. So what can you do if cheese is high on your list of life's priorities? Here are some tips:

► Try lower-fat cheeses such as cottage cheese, ricotta and feta.

► Eat fuller-fat cheeses in smaller amounts.

► Make your fuller-fat soft cheeses go a long way by eating them with low-fat crackers or fruit or celery sticks.

► Grating hard cheeses will make them go further.

► Go for a small amount of a strongly flavoured cheese, such as a Stilton, rather than eating larger amounts of milder-tasting cheeses.

NUTS

Peanuts are actually a legume, but we generally refer to them as nuts. Nuts, peanuts and peanut butter are mostly fat, so should we avoid them?

As we have seen in this book, there are bad fats but there are also good fats. In 2002 a very interesting piece of research on nuts was published in the prestigious *Journal of the American Medical Association* (JAMA). Entitled 'Nut and peanut butter consumption and risk of type-2 diabetes in women', it showed that women who ate at least 140g (5oz) of peanuts and peanut butter a week reduced their risk of developing type-2 diabetes by 21 per cent compared to those who rarely or never ate them. The research also found that women who often ate tree nuts, such as almonds, walnuts, cashew nuts, pecan nuts and pistachio nuts, reduced their risk of type-2 diabetes by 27 per cent compared to women who rarely ate them.

Won't nuts make you put on weight, though? In a major piece of research on over 80,000 American nurses over 16 years, scientists found that women who ate the most nuts tended to weigh a bit less and have a lower BMI than the others.

Nuts and peanuts are rich in the healthy kinds of fats – monounsaturated and polyunsaturated – and both are good sources of antioxidants, protein, magnesium and fibre. They also have a low GI and have good effects on cholesterol and triglyceride levels. Research shows that the more nuts we eat the less our risk of coronary heart disease. If you want to avoid heart disease and diabetes, eat more nuts, peanuts and peanut butter instead of fatty meats and refined grains. But, of course, remember that everything should be in moderation.

Here is a list of the saturated fat and total fat content of some popular nuts:

THE SATURATED FAT CONTENT OF NUTS

Nut, 25g (1oz) portion	Saturated fat (g)	Total fat (g)
Almonds, dry-roasted	1.4g	14.6g
Brazil nuts	4.6g	19g
Cashew nuts	2.6g	13.2g
Chestnuts	trace	0.3g
Coconut, dried	16g	18.3g

▶

Nut, 25g (1oz) portion	Saturated fat (g)	Total fat (g)
Hazelnuts	1.4g	18.8g
Macadamia nuts	3.1g	21g
Mixed nuts, oil-roasted	2.5g	16g
Pecan nuts	1.5g	18.3g
Peanuts, dry-roasted	2g	14g
Peanuts, oil-roasted	2.5g	16g
Peanuts, boiled (shelled)	1g	6g
Peanuts, Spanish, raw	2g	14g
Peanuts, chocolate coated (10 nuts)	6g	13g
Pine nuts	2.2g	14.3g
Pistachio nuts	1.7g	137g
Walnuts	1g	16g

You will find my recommended quantities of nuts in the snack sections of the Daily Menus in Chapters 19 and 22.

Chapter Twelve

SUPPLEMENTS

ARE SUPPLEMENTS WORTH TAKING, or are they a waste of time? Doctors disagree on this. A lot of the medical press pooh-poohs supplements, but at medical seminars I am always surprised at the number of eminent specialists who secretly admit to taking them. Let's look at a few different types of supplements.

VITAMIN PILLS

I admit to taking a variety of supplements. These include:

B vitamins, especially vitamin B_{12} and folic acid, which I take because there is evidence that high blood levels of homocysteine (in the metabolism of which the B-vitamins, folate and B_{12}, play a key role) may be a risk factor for Alzheimer's disease and coronary heart disease.

There is a considerable difference in death rates from heart disease and stroke between northern and southern European countries. A key difference is the higher consumption of fruit and vegetables in the south. It used to be thought that this protective effect of fruit and vegetables was due to antioxidants. But fruit and vegetables are also one of the main dietary sources of folate, which probably has a beneficial effect on the lining of arteries. Taking folic acid supplements over many years may also substantially reduce the risk of breast and bowel cancer.

Selenium is important for the body's immune system, which is vital to fight infection, and it seems to be a key nutrient in stopping HIV progressing to AIDS. It is needed for sperm motility and may reduce the risk of miscarriage. Selenium deficiency has been linked to depression. Selenium and vitamin E may be helpful in reducing heart disease and stroke as well as cancer risk. In particular, research suggests that high selenium and vitamin E intake may lower the risk of prostate cancer. There is some evidence that vitamin E may also be helpful in Alzheimer's disease.

Vitamin D In the UK, about 80 per cent of us are deficient in vitamin D. The reason for this isn't hard to find. Lack of sunshine might be a clue.

Fish oils The evidence first reported 20 years ago from the Greenland Inuit population suggested that fatty fish and fish oils contained substances that reduced the incidence of coronary heart disease. These substances – omega-3 fatty acids, which we have discussed earlier – were found in early clinical trials to reduce platelet stickiness and to lower the levels of triglycerides by as much as 35 per cent. More recent trials have found that omega-3 fatty acids also appear to reduce the risk of abnormal heart rhythms and sudden cardiac death and modestly reduce atherosclerosis plaque formation and high blood pressure. Omega-3 fish oils may also reduce the risk of stroke. Omega-3 oils are good for a baby's brain and nerve development in late pregnancy. For a more in-depth look at omega-3s see the previous chapter.

Vitamins are also known to help reduce inflammation which, as we have seen earlier, plays an important role in why so many of us struggle to lose weight.

How much should we take?

This is difficult to answer. There hasn't been enough research to give definitive answers, but, as a guide, let me tell you what I take each day:

Supplement	Dosage
Multivitamin–mineral	1 tablet
plus	
Folic acid	800mg
Vitamin D	800iu
Omega-3 (EPA) fish oils	1,000mg × 2 (but see below)

The B vitamins and selenium listed above are included in a good-quality multivitamin–mineral. You can buy these from your high-street shops and I suggest you stick to the recommended daily amounts (RDAs) as specified on the labels.

Before taking any supplements, remember the following two important points:

1. These are *supplements*. That means that they are to be taken *as well as* a healthy balanced diet with its minimum of five portions of fruit and vegetables a day – not instead of.

2. Do please first check with your doctor that it is OK for you to take them.

Omega-3 supplements

The case for the benefits of omega-3 supplements is far from clear-cut. Recent research has cast doubt on the accepted belief that omega-3 supplements reduce the risk if cardiovascular disease and prostate cancer. Indeed, some research strongly suggests that omega-3 supplements may actually increase the risk of prostate cancer, although at the same time they may reduce the risk of colon cancer; however, there seems to be a consensus currently that omega-3 supplementation probably reduces the risk of intraductal carcinoma, which is the commonest form of breast cancer.

Prebiotics and probiotics

See Chapter 4 for a discussion of prebiotics and probiotics and page 138 for my recommended dietary supplements.

Chapter Thirteen

HOW TO LOSE WEIGHT WITHOUT REALLY DIETING

I T MUST BE EVERY SLIMMER'S DREAM to learn how to lose weight without really dieting – and that was the title of my first slimming book. It's a 'no-diet' diet. With the exception of sugar, which is best to avoid if we can, we can eat pretty well whatever we like. The important point is that we eat a little less of everything that we are used to. Many of the popular diets fail to work in the long term because of limiting foods, a boring selection of meal suggestions or weight gain returning once the target weight is reached. So what makes for a successful sustainable slimming approach? What, then, are its essential 'ingredients'? We've looked at these earlier in this book, but just to recap:

1. We must lose weight. That's obvious really, but it's amazing how many slimming methods don't result in weight loss.

2. We shouldn't eventually regain the weight we've lost.

3. We shouldn't experience hunger and other unpleasant sensations.

4. Our diet should be a healthy well-balanced one with all the essential nutrients.

5. Losing weight mustn't be antisocial. Turning down food that has been lovingly prepared by someone else won't make us too popular.

6. Losing weight should be pleasant. If our diet contains mainly foods that we dislike and doesn't allow us to eat our favourite foods, we aren't likely to stick with it.

7. Losing weight must be simple. We don't really want to go around with calculators to work out exactly what we can eat mouthful by mouthful.

8. Our slimming programme must be *sustainable* in the long term.

If we apply these points to well-known diets, most fail for one or more reasons. The freedom of 'how to lose weight without really dieting', which scores perfectly on all the points above, makes it very attractive. It really is the commonsense approach to eating less. But be careful here. We're talking about eating a little less, *not* a lot less. One slice of bread instead of two, one or two potatoes instead of three or four. With two exceptions, which we'll look at shortly, we don't have to make any significant changes to our food or drink. We can even eat cakes and chocolates, provided we don't have them every day and make them an occasional treat.

The two exceptions I mentioned above are very simple and not a hardship. First, whenever possible, we should try to use a less fattening method of preparing or cooking food; for example, a portion of grilled bacon saves 100 calories compared to the same portion fried – and it tastes much better because it is less greasy! A non-stick frying pan is really handy if you like fried foods, because you can then fry most foods in their own fat. You can fry an egg, for example, without any butter or oil and save 40 calories. You can pre-fry vegetables without added oil or fat, so that if you want a minced meat dish with vegetables, you first heat the meat slowly and then add the vegetables. There are so many other ways to save calories; for example, with a steak and kidney pie, why not have a single crust on top rather than a double crust? And do you really need to thicken the gravy with calorific flour?

The second exception is this: try to cut out as much sugar from food and drinks as you can. Apart from the calories – 30 of them – each teaspoon of sugar has no nutritional value at all. If you have a 'sweet tooth', why not use artificial sweeteners? These are available in tablet, liquid and powder forms and so can be sprinkled over breakfast cereal and can be used in cooking. Some people object to their taste at first, but it is surprising how quickly most of us soon acquire the taste for them if we try (see also the box below).

It is really important to avoid all hidden forms of sugar, for example in soft drinks. Use low-calorie versions and you save at least 70 calories a glass. And some low-calorie drinks, especially tonic water, are more appealing. In fact, when you feel tempted to put food in your mouth and it isn't time for a meal, why not pour yourself a low-calorie tonic water or lemonade? Make a real 'meal' of it by adding ice cubes and a slice of lemon and even some Angostura bitters. Sit down and enjoy it, savour it, sip by sip. Although some parts of the popular press have said that low-calorie drinks can actually contribute to weight gain – the so-called 'diet cola belly' – I have seen no good evidence in any reputable scientific journal that supports that view.

ARTIFICIAL SWEETENERS

The internet is a wonderful resource. You can find out everything there is to know about almost anything. One of its uses is to find out more about health issues. But there is a downside: many health web pages are written or hosted by people with little or no scientific training or by others who espouse ideas and theories that have little or no scientific basis. A prime example is the enormous nonsense written about the supposed dangers of artificial sweeteners, which have been targeted by the 'anti' lobby ever since the 1970s, when saccharin was condemned because it was linked to bladder cancer in laboratory rats. The flaw in the lobby's argument was that the doses of saccharin were many thousand times those used by humans to sweeten their food and drink.

The US National Cancer Institute has found no scientific evidence that any of the artificial sweeteners approved for use in the US cause cancer or other serious health problems. This has been confirmed by a wealth of other research, which has shown that artificial sweeteners are safe in the quantities used in human consumption. The National Cancer Institute has published a fact sheet in which the key messages are that there is no clear evidence that the artificial sweeteners available commercially in the US (and UK) are associated with a cancer risk in humans. Studies have been conducted on the safety of several artificial sweeteners, including saccharin, aspartame, acesulfame potassium, sucralose, neotame and cyclamate.

If you prefer to eat natural foods, you could try xylitol (derived from silver birch) and stevia (derived from the leaf of the plant *Stevia rebaudiana*). Both are easily available from health-food shops. Note, however, that xylitol can sometimes cause bloating, flatulence and diarrhoea and is probably best limited to small amounts.

Syrup in tinned fruit is another source of hidden sugar, so always buy tinned fruit without the highly calorific syrup.

HOW TO CUT CORNERS

Here are a few examples of how we can easily save calories by eating just a little less. Take breakfast: do you fancy cornflakes, bacon and eggs, toast and coffee? Let's look at each of these:

Cornflakes, 25g (1oz)	100 calories
Milk, 140g (5oz)	95 calories
Sugar, 2 tsp	60 calories
Total	**255 calories**

By eating just a little less:

Cornflakes, 20g (⅔oz)	70 calories
Milk, 85g (3oz)	55 calories
Sugar, 1 tsp	30 calories
Total	**155 calories**

And then by substituting low-calorie versions where possible, including skimmed milk (which is an easily acquired taste – honestly!):

Cornflakes, 20g (⅔oz)	70 calories
Skimmed milk, 85g (3oz)	30 calories
Artificial sweetener	0 calories
Total	**100 calories**

We've reduced the number of calories from 255 to 100 – a saving of 155 calories. And the chances are that we'll barely notice that we're eating less or that we're using artificial sweetener and skimmed milk. (By the way, I'm not advocating that we eat corn-flakes. As cereals go, there are many others that I think are better for slimmers, but I'm simply using them as an example, because that's how many people start their day.)

Now, bacon and eggs:

Bacon (streaky), fried, 2 rashers	170 calories
Egg fried in oil or butter	135 calories
Total	**305 calories**

Compared with:

Bacon (streaky), grilled, 1 rasher	40 calories
Egg fried in its own fat in a non-stick pan	95 calories
Total	**135 calories**

By eating a little less bacon (cooked to be more crispy because it is grilled) plus an egg we save 170 calories.

Now for toast and marmalade. The important point is to spread butter (or margarine) and marmalade (or jam) very, very thinly – just enough to give us a taste:

Toast, 2 slices	145 calories
Butter, 15g (½oz) per slice	225 calories
Marmalade, 15g (½oz) per slice	75 calories
Total	**445 calories**

Compare that with eating just one slice of toast, using low-calorie margarine – and most of us won't even notice the difference in taste, sandwiched between the toast and the marmalade – and spreading the margarine very thinly:

Toast, 1 slice	70 calories
Low-calorie margarine, 8g (¼oz) per slice	25 calories
Marmalade, 8g (¼oz) per slice	20 calories
Total	**115 calories**

Let's suppose we want to be really 'naughty' and have fried fish and chips for lunch:

Fried haddock, 175g (6oz)	635 calories
Chips, 5oz (140g)	435 calories
Total	**1,070 calories**

By using larger chips (which soak up less oil, because the total surface area is smaller) and grilling them, rather than frying, and with the fish grilled, we can save a huge number of calories:

Grilled haddock, 115g (4oz)	190 calories
Chips (large), 85g (3oz)	115 calories
Total	**305 calories**

An afternoon cup of tea or coffee:

Tea (or coffee), 5fl oz (150ml)	0 calories
Milk, 25ml (1fl oz)	20 calories
Sugar, 2 tsp	60 calories
Total	**85 calories**

Compare that with:

Tea (or coffee), 5fl oz (150ml)	0 calories
Skimmed milk, 25ml (1fl oz)	10 calories
Artificial sweetener	0 calories
Total	**10 calories**

Supper:

Tomato soup (cream), 280g (10oz)	420 calories

Compare that with:

Tomato soup (cream), 175g (6oz)	250 calories

and:

Tomato soup, low-calorie, 175g (6oz)	40 calories

Followed by:

Hamburgers, medium size, frozen, fried, 2	320 calories
Potatoes, mashed, 140g (5oz)	170 calories
Mushrooms, fried, 55g (2oz)	65 calories
Tomatoes, fried, 115g (4oz)	80 calories
Total	**635 calories**

With smaller portions and grilling the hamburgers instead of frying them, and eating baked instead of mashed potato (which, incidentally, preserves more of its vitamin C):

Hamburgers, medium size, frozen, grilled, 1½	135 calories
Baked potato (no added butter or cream)	70 calories
Mushrooms, grilled, 45g (1½oz)	5 calories
Tomatoes, grilled, 85g (3oz)	10 calories
Total	**220 calories**

By the way, I'm certainly not suggesting that we should have fish and chips for lunch and hamburgers in the evening! I'm just using them to illustrate some important principles. Nor am I suggesting that mashed or baked potatoes are ideal for weight control. I'm just using them to illustrate how a popular vegetable accompaniment can be made less calorific. The best potato option is new potatoes, which are low-GI.

Finally:

Apple pie, 140g (5oz)	270 calories
Cream, 55g (2oz)	465 calories
Total	**735 calories**

Compare this with:

Apple pie, 85g (3oz)	160 calories
Cream, 25g (1oz)	230 calories
Total	**390 calories**

Assuming four cups of tea or coffee a day, the total savings on the examples I have quoted for one day amount to 2,830 calories which would result in a true weight loss (that is, fat loss) of about 13 ounces; that's almost 1 pound (or just under ½kg). And this is without starving ourselves or having to go particularly hungry and without significant changes to our food.

Chapter Fourteen

EATING OUT

THERE WILL ALWAYS BE THE day that every person who's trying to lose weight dreads, and I don't mean Christmas or holidays, which, of course, may present a challenge. What I have in mind is the day we are invited to go out for a meal in a restaurant. At home we can control what we cook and eat. But in a restaurant, what do we do? My earlier book *How to Lose Weight Without Really Dieting* assured me that I don't need to diet as long as I eat healthily. But has the chef read that book? Is the food in this restaurant healthy? When we look at the menu, our first glance suggests we might have a challenge. Our heart sinks, then we look at the door and think, *Should we go now before we've even started?* Or do we say to ourselves, 'Blow losing weight, I'll gorge myself for once'?

The good news is that we don't have to do either. It's quite feasible to make healthy food choices virtually wherever we are. We just need to remember a few basic principles:

1. Eat any kind of meat as long as it is lean.

2. Eat any grilled fish, seafood or poultry.

3. Choose the healthiest cooking methods: grilled, steamed, boiled, roasted or stir-fried.

4. Ask for sauces to be served on one side so that you control how much you eat.

5. Eat most fruit and vegetables, but when it comes to potatoes ask for small new ones if at all possible. Of course, the odd one or two potatoes once in a while when we eat out will do us no harm, but try to avoid chips, baked or mashed potatoes, as these have a higher GI. New potatoes are a better option.

6. Eat salads liberally. Ask for a light dressing or a little olive oil. Balsamic vinegar is one of my favourites.

7. Don't stuff yourself on bread. In fact, it's best to avoid it altogether unless it is wholegrain or sourdough. Again, as with potatoes, the odd slice even of white bread occasionally will do us no harm. Go very easy on the butter though; it's better to avoid it altogether if you can.

8. Don't feel that you necessarily have to have a conventional starter, a main and a dessert. In most restaurants we can ask for two starters followed by, say, a salad. The portions are likely to be smaller and therefore less calorific.

9. If you really can't resist a rich dessert, how about sharing one between two people?

10. Don't be shy about leaving food on your plate. To the inevitable 'Didn't you like it?' from the waiter you can smile sweetly and explain that you are watching your figure and ask the waiter to pass your compliments on to the chef.

11. Try not to arrive at the restaurant starving hungry. If you do, you are bound to over-eat.

12. Have a light, healthy low-GI snack, such as a portion of fruit, before you go. My favourite is a couple of tablespoons of rolled oats, which I eat without milk. (You will find a selection of snacks in the Daily Menus in Chapters 19 and 22.)

CHINESE

It comes as a surprise to many people that Chinese food presents few challenges, because it has plenty of vegetables and it is low in fat. If we stick to lean meat, seafood and vegetables, all of which are available in a wide range of dishes, and go for stir-fried in preference to deep-fried food, we won't go far wrong.

Choose:

▶ Clear soups, such as won ton, hot-and-sour.

▶ Stir-fries with lean meat, poultry, seafood, vegetables and tofu.

▶ Steamed fish.

▶ Vegetables.

▶ Noodles with chicken, seafood or vegetable lo mein (in which the noodles are stir-fried with the other ingredients).

▶ Chop suey (but no fried noodles).

▶ Chow mein (but no fried noodles).

▶ Sauces: black bean, mustard, oyster, Szechuan.

It's a good idea, when eating noodles, to keep the portion size small in favour of more vegetables.

Avoid:

▶ White rice other than one or two tablespoonfuls. Ask for long-grain rice, although the chances of getting this in a Chinese restaurant are slim, in which case opt for Oriental noodles (egg, rice or mung bean).

Ask for:

▶ Sauces to be served on one side, so that you can control how much you eat.

ITALIAN

Moderation is the key for Italian food. Pizzas are fine as long as they are thin crust with a minimum of cheese toppings (go for vegetable toppings instead). Cappuccino is also OK, but ask for skinny cappuccino (that is, one made with skimmed or semi-skimmed milk).

Choose:

▶ Pasta, but ask for it to be *al dente* and eat a small portion – about a handful – as a starter or a side order.

▶ Avoid cheese or cream sauces. Instead, go for tomato-based or seafood-based sauces.

▶ Vegetable soup (minestrone) or bean-based soup (pasta fagioli).

▶ Lean beef.

▶ Veal (but no breadcrumbs).

► Grilled chicken.

► Seafood.

Avoid:

► Bread, unless it is semolina bread, and even then only one small piece.

FRENCH

This can be quite a challenge because of all the butter, cream and cheese, not to mention French bread, which has just about the highest GI of all breads. Remember, however, that in France people traditionally eat small portions, so practise portion control, and it's also worth going for the less creamy dishes to keep calories down.

Choose:

► Consommé.

► Chicken and fish Provençale (with tomato sauce).

► Chicken and meat stews (with tomato or wine sauces).

► Bouillabaisse (seafood stew).

► Ratatouille (vegetable stew).

► Steamed or poached chicken, seafood and vegetables.

► Grilled meats without sauce, or with the sauce on the side.

► Salads.

► Plenty of accompanying vegetables.

Avoid:

▶ French bread.

INDIAN

As with Chinese cuisine, it surprises many that Indian cuisine is slimmer-friendly. Pulses, chicken, fish, vegetables and yoghurt are all healthy options. Basmati rice is also good. The downside with Indian food is that often a lot of fat is used for frying, and many sauces have a heavy ghee (clarified butter) base, so we need to ask for as little fat and butter to be used as possible.

Choose:

▶ Lentil or bean soups.

▶ Biryanis (made with basmati rice).

▶ Curries made with chicken, seafood or vegetables (but avoid those made with coconut).

▶ Chicken or lamb kebabs.

▶ Tandoori chicken or fish (where the main ingredient is marinated in yoghurt and then baked).

▶ Chicken or shrimp vindaloo.

JAPANESE

The Japanese have a long life expectancy, and so far no one has satisfactorily explained why this is so. Until recently it was thought to be to do with their food, which, with the exception of sticky white rice, teriyaki sauce and tinned lychees, was regarded as very healthy. Of course, rice-based sushi is a staple component of the Japanese diet, so in recent years the diet is no longer viewed as being particularly healthy, and we have yet to find the reason why Japanese people living in Japan (as opposed to in the West) are generally so healthy. Unless you're Japanese, it's probably best to regard a visit to a Japanese restaurant as a very occasional treat.

THAI

Although Thai food is delicious and some of it is quite healthy, you need to be aware of some unhealthy choices. These include: deep-fried spring rolls and dumplings, especially when served with salty, fatty or sugary sauces; curry dishes with coconut milk, which is high in saturated fats; peanut sauce; and satay, which is a combination of coconut milk and peanut-oil-fried rice. Always choose small portions. Sharing dishes can be a way of keeping portions within limits.

MEXICAN

Unfortunately, Mexican cuisine can be challenging for people wanting to lose weight. The food is mainly high in starch and fat and low in fruit and vegetables, leading to an overload of both calories and carbs.

Choose:

▶ Grilled chicken and seafood.

▶ Salads.

▶ Beans.

▶ Fajitas, burritos, tacos and quesadillas made with wholewheat tortillas.

Avoid:

▶ High-starch, high-fat foods (including chips) – they are denser in calories than they are in nutrients.

▶ Limit cheese and soured cream, or ask if low-fat varieties are available.

TAKEAWAYS

What is the best way to approach takeaways? The short answer is: try to avoid them, except as a very occasional special treat. Their fat content is generally high and the bread and rolls used, as in hamburgers, have very high GIs.

Chapter Fifteen

THINKING LIGHT – THE 30 RULES FOR GETTING SLIM AND STAYING THERE

RECOGNISING THE CUES THAT make us eat when we're not actually hungry and handling how we deal with those cues is extremely important if we want to lose weight while still mainly eating the foods we enjoy.

The only useful cue to eat is hunger. Unfortunately, however, we've conditioned ourselves to respond to other cues: habit, boredom, anger and so on. The trouble is that these cues are irrelevant and inappropriate when it comes to our body's needs for food. We've lost the ability to recognise and respond to the disappearance of hunger, which should be the cue to stop eating. Animals that live in the wild rarely become overweight. A lion will go without food for two or three days. Only when it feels hungry will it hunt and kill to provide a meal. And it will stop eating once it is no longer hungry, even if there is still some meat left on the carcass. The lion is using hunger as its control for when to start and when to stop eating. Similarly, a breast-fed baby will suck only when he or she is hungry and then stops sucking when no longer hungry.

Let's look at some of our **eating cues**. Some are good, but most are bad. We'll look at how we can discourage the undesirable ones and how we can encourage the useful ones by adopting a set of useful rules.

First, let's focus on when we buy food. FACT: people who shop after a meal when they are not hungry buy less food.

RULE 1 Shop for food as soon as possible after a meal rather than when your stomach is empty.

Our minds are easily persuaded to buy colourful and attractive foods and to buy foods that we did not intend to buy.

RULE 2 Make a list of the foods you intend to buy.

Keep that list in your hand while shopping, and stick rigidly to it.

RULE 3 Take sufficient money only for the food on your list, and no more.

I once had a patient who, when she was out, could never walk past a shop that sold food without going in and buying something. I told her that if she was not out for the specific purpose of buying food she should leave her purse at home.

RULE 4 List the shops where you intend to buy food and don't go into other ones.

Planning our meals each day is very important. It's not so much what we eat at these meals but when we eat. The idea is to satisfy our hunger at proper mealtimes and to avoid between-meal snacking other than very small ones. Also, skipped meals tend to cause excessive hunger, which in turn leads to gorging. Very often the person who only has a cup of coffee for breakfast and no lunch will be so hungry by the evening that they will eat more food for the evening meal than they might otherwise have done if they had eaten three meals (when the total calorie intake might well have been less than that in one large meal a day).

Rule 5 Avoid excessive hunger by having regular, planned meals. Plan these meals daily and stick to your plan.

One or two healthy snacks a day are fine, if you find you need them. (You'll find some suggestions below and in Chapters 19 and 22.) It's amazing, though, how much food we eat when we're *not really hungry*. And it's this extra food that is often the reason why we find it difficult to control our weight. It's essential to remember Rule 6 below.

Some light, healthy snacks

► slice of low-fat cheese

► a piece of fruit

► a bowl of cherries

► 4 dried apricots

► a carrot

► celery stick stuffed with any low-fat cheese e.g. cottage cheese, Laughing Cow light cheese

► celery stick with hummus

► 5 Brazil nuts

► 8 cashew nuts

► 10 peanuts, unsalted

► 8 walnuts

► 15 pistachio nuts

► 1oz flax seeds or sesame seeds

► 2 tablespoons of rolled oats

RULE 6 Eat only if and when you're hungry. If you're not hungry don't eat.

If we have three meals a day, each of which need only be fairly light, we're almost certain to feel at least a little hungry at mealtimes. But using hunger as an eating control doesn't end there. We have to stop eating when we're no longer hungry – something we'll look at shortly.

RULE 7 Do not overdraw on your calories in advance.

It's very tempting to 'overdraw' on our calories in advance, so that perhaps we think it's OK to have a mid-morning snack by saying to ourselves that it can be instead of our lunchtime dessert. The chances are that when it comes to lunch we'll still have our dessert. It's probably better to go without dessert at lunchtime in favour of a teatime snack, although having snacks at all is dangerous when we're trying to control our weight, unless we choose very wisely and follow the suggestions I make for healthy snacks in the Daily Menus in Chapters 19 and 22.

It's so important that our choice of food isn't too limited. It's no use following a diet that's so strict that some of the ingredients or dishes on the diet wouldn't be available on a restaurant menu, for example. We must always have reasonable alternatives. This is why my principle of 'how to lose weight without really dieting' works so well, because, within reason, you can eat what you want.

RULE 8 Always follow a diet plan that offers you alternatives.

That's the big plus with the principles I promote in this book.

RULE 9 Make low-calorie foods more interesting by cooking with spices and using imaginative low-calorie garnishes.

Low-calorie foods can be boring, but we can make them more appealing by dressing them up with low-calorie additions such as fresh parsley, coriander or mint, and using garlic and spices in cooking. We can really let our imagination run riot here and add some flavour combinations from around the world to brighten up our meals.

The next rules look at **eating behaviour during mealtimes**. This is the most important area of all, because there are many opportunities for modifying our eating behaviour.

RULE 10 When at home, always eat in the same room.

Eating should be an activity with its own time and place, just like any other activity. We play squash on a squash court, we swim in a swimming pool, we drive a car on a road, we sleep in our bedroom and we wash in our bathroom. So, we eat in our 'eating room', usually our kitchen or dining room – at least when we're at home.

RULE 11 Always eat in the same place in the one room in which you have your meals.

Always eat while sitting on the *same chair at the same position* at the table. This space becomes our personal eating area.

RULE 12 Eat only when you are sitting at a dining table.

RULE 13 Never put anything in your mouth (except a toothbrush) while you are standing.

Let's now get back to the most important point:

Eat only if and when you're hungry (which is Rule 6).

Whether or not we're hungry is not just a once-and-for-all decision we take at the start of a meal. Just as hunger is the cue to eat, so the lack or disappearance of hunger is the cue to stop eating.

But we can only decide we're no longer hungry, and therefore that we should stop eating if, during the course of the meal, we periodically ask ourselves, 'Am I still hungry?'

RULE 14 While eating, periodically ask yourself, 'Am I still hungry?'

If your honest answer is no, stop eating. It takes 15–20 minutes for the brain to register that the stomach is full, so eat slowly to allow your brain to recognise that you are no longer hungry.

Ignoring this rule is an important reason why most people become overweight and have difficulty losing weight. Of course, for many of us, it goes against the grain to leave food on the plate. We've been brought up to think it's simply wrong. In a restaurant, it's a waste of money to leave all that delicious food Or is it?

One of my patients told me her challenge was eating at friends' homes. She was always far too polite ever to refuse anything. A doting mother can also be a challenge to a slimmer – a good appetite is supposed to be a sign of good health. If we refuse food fondly cooked by our mother, galloping paranoia sets in and she assumes something must be wrong with her cooking. Incidentally, I was photographed for a previous slimming book by a royal photographer who told me that older members of the Royal Family follow Rule 14 very strictly – only two or three mouthfuls at each of the many courses, the rest of the food being left on the plates. They pace the meal so that enough hunger is left for each succeeding course. The result? They can enjoy even the dessert without worrying about their weight. Several A-listers adopt a variation on this rule when eating out: draw a line down the middle of every plateful of solid food with a knife and eat just half the food.

RULE 15 During meals, focus on eating and avoid distractions.

To use Rule 14 we obviously need to be completely aware throughout the meal of just how hungry we are. We have to be focused with no distractions, such as reading at the table, watching television or solving a crossword puzzle.

RULE 16 Always use a knife, fork or spoon for *all* solid food.

Another way to help ensure that we remain focused during meals is to make sure we never eat food mindlessly and, therefore, when we might not even be hungry. A great way to be sure of this is always to eat solid food with a knife, fork or spoon. Never, never use your fingers. Using cutlery makes us think much more about the fact that we are eating, whereas putting food into our mouth with our fingers just doesn't seem quite so much like eating. It's amazing how many peanuts can disappear down our throats without our noticing! I have patients who even eat a sandwich with a knife and fork. If we make it an open sandwich, it doesn't seem ridiculous.

RULE 17 Limit the time you allow yourself for each meal.

Time-limiting and delaying strategies are very useful ways of controlling how much we eat. An obvious strategy is to say we'll give ourselves just 10 minutes for breakfast (for example), 20 minutes for lunch and 25 minutes for supper or dinner. By the way, this strategy works only if we don't eat faster in order to consume more food!

RULE 18 Make it a little more difficult to get food at mealtimes.

Another delaying strategy is to make it a little more difficult to get food at mealtimes; for example, at breakfast we could toast only one slice of bread (or even just half a slice) at a time. When we've eaten that, then we can go back to the toaster and put in another slice of bread and wait by the toaster until the toast is ready. This is likely to make us feel we can't be bothered to eat several slices of toast. One of my patients keeps her toaster upstairs. Every time she wants another slice of toast she has to go upstairs to make it and then she brings it downstairs to eat it. Perhaps that's a bit extreme.

RULE 19 Put down your knife, fork or spoon for a minute or so between mouthfuls.

An interesting fact is that often the more quickly we eat food, the more we eat. People who never put down their knives and forks and who busy themselves by cutting up and preparing their next mouthful while still chewing food tend to eat quickly and therefore eat more of it. A good delaying strategy is to put down your knife and fork on your plate between mouthfuls for a minute so.

RULE 20 Cut up your food into as many small pieces as you can.

Another delaying tactic is to cut up your food into many small pieces. This makes the plate look as if there is more food on it than there actually is, and cutting up food takes up time, which leaves you with less time to actually eat it.

RULE 21 Serve your food on a small plate and spread the food evenly over the plate.

Make the strategy in Rule 20 even more effective by using a small plate and spreading the food evenly over it. This makes it look as if there is more food on the plate than there actually is.

RULE 22 Serve yourself small, measured quantities of food rather than helping yourself ad lib.

When serving ourselves it's a good idea to use small, measured quantities – say, one or two tablespoons of mashed potato, for example – rather than helping ourselves ad lib from a large serving bowl.

RULE 23 Do not keep serving dishes on the table while you eat.

When you take the serving dishes off the table you remove the temptation to help yourself to further helpings of food after you've begun eating. It's a good idea to serve on the kitchen work-top and not bother with serving bowls other than salad.

RULE 24 Chew each mouthful for as long as possible.

The 19th-century British Prime Minister, William Gladstone, is said to have chewed each mouthful until it turned to water – a great delaying tactic!

RULE 25 Count and try to reduce the number of mouthfuls you take.

Count how many mouthfuls you eat in a period of, say, two or three minutes, then reduce the number of mouthfuls, so that you eat more slowly.

RULE 26 Swallow all the food from each mouthful before putting any more food into your mouth.

This also extends the period of time you eat and gives you the chance to properly enjoy it.

One patient told me how she discovered how quickly she ate. She put her table under a wall-mounted mirror and watched herself eating. She was appalled by the sight of herself gobbling her food, scarcely pausing to breathe between mouthfuls, and just shovelling her food into her mouth. The mirror ploy is really useful.

RULE 27 After finishing your meal, dispose of any leftovers immediately.

Even after we've told ourselves we're no longer hungry, it can be very tempting to pick at food as long as it's in front of us. Children's leftovers are a good example – many mothers pick at these.

RULE 28 Leave the table as soon as you've finished eating.

If you can, leave the table between courses!

RULE 29 Let others, especially children (if old enough), get their own healthy snacks, such as nuts, from the cupboard, and put the chocolate out of sight in a high cupboard out of reach. Make chocolate-eating an occasional treat that you, and your family, plan and enjoy.

We must try to avoid putting ourselves into direct contact with foods that may tempt us, and it's worth planning ahead to eat small amounts of foods that are not healthy to eat every day. A couple of cubes of 85-per-cent-cocoa-solids chocolate, for example, can satisfy your chocolate craving and can actually be beneficial for your health when eaten occasionally (but certainly not every day).

Many of the rules I've described so far mean that we eat less food, while at the same time – and this is so important – we actually *increase our enjoyment* of food. I often hear from people who fail to lose weight: 'I enjoy my food too much.' If that sounds familiar, think for a moment about the difference between a gourmet and a gourmand. A gourmand is a glutton who eats anything and everything. A gourmet, on the other hand, is highly selective about what he or she eats. A gourmet is a connoisseur who enjoys food, not because of how much there is but because of its flavour, smell, texture and appearance. A gourmet eats less food than a gourmand but enjoys it more.

Next time you eat in a restaurant, notice how other people eat. The fast eaters eat more food and are often overweight, whereas the slow, thoughtful eaters are usually slim. Enjoying food is all about quality, not quantity. As Sir Walter A. Raleigh (not the Elizabethan, but the late-19th- and early-20th-century writer) wrote in *Laughter from a Cloud*:

Eat slowly: only men in rags
And gluttons old in sin
Mistake themselves for carpet bags
And tumble victuals in.

Let's not be carpet bags!

Unfortunately, no amount of rules will be enough for some people who want to lose weight – their motivation and

---

SMALL TEMPTATIONS

If we feel tempted to eat chocolates, limit how many we have. Leaving an open box in front of us is fatal – it's no surprise how easily the chocolates disappear into our mouths before we even realise it! A good idea is to take the chocolate (or chocolates) that we're going to eat out of the box and then put the box away out of sight *before* we start to eat any of the chocolates. We can savour each chocolate (which, after all, we're eating only for its taste). We can nibble the chocolate, bit by bit, roll it around our mouth with our tongue, and try not to let our mind be distracted away from enjoying the chocolate.

This is how we can get maximum pleasure from perhaps only one chocolate, and there will be no need to eat our way through a boxful.

If eating a chocolate is something that only occurs to you when you see a box, or if you know that there's a box in the cupboard, it's best not keep chocolates in the home at all. What isn't there can't be eaten! In fact, it's a good idea to avoid all snackable foods in the home and keep only those foods that take time to prepare.

determination seem to weaken from time to time. For those of us who fall into this group, some of the following strategies might be helpful:

A nylon cord This can be useful when we've already lost weight and then find ourselves starting to put weight back on again. The idea started with ultra-slim photographic models who tied a thin gold chain around their waists. If the chain became tighter they knew they were putting on weight. Fortunately, a nylon cord works just as well without burning a hole in your pocket! Tie the nylon cord around your waist. The cord should be fairly thin (about 2mm/⅛in) so that it doesn't show through your clothes. Tie it sufficiently tightly so that when you sit it causes a white (but not red) line to be visible in your skin. When you lie down it shouldn't cause an indentation. Keep the cord on at all times, even when in the bath. Every few days, as you lose weight, you tighten the cord a little more. If, while you're still trying to lose weight, or after you've reached your target weight, the cord becomes tighter, you know that your weight has started to creep up again. Don't forget, incidentally, that if you are a woman, fluid retention may cause an increase in your waist pre-menstrually, so do allow for this.

A notebook When you feel an irresistible urge to eat when you're not hungry, a useful strategy is write down your thoughts before you eat. Just doing this may well stop you from eating. (See also about writing a food diary on page 176.)

A camera Another strategy is to photograph the food you want to eat but know you shouldn't. Doing this may make you think twice about eating it.

A slim-buddy These are a great idea. In fact, for a time I was consultant to a website devoted to slim-buddies. If you have a friend, or friends, who are trying to lose weight, why not agree to telephone each other when feeling desperate about the temptation to eat? Forming your own self-help group might be enormously helpful and motivating during those times when you find yourself weakening,

I'd like to stress that most of us are unlikely to need these added strategies, but I mention them for those people who might find them helpful.

And now we come to the last of the Rules. One of the slimmer's big enemies is boredom. Eating just for something to do, the dreaded snacking impulse, happens when we're bored. For those of us who often feel bored, it's worth spending time looking at our lifestyle; for example, at the end of the day do you slump in a chair with a box of chocolates by your side as you watch TV? Do you automatically head for the fridge and look for goodies? If so, try to think up alternative activities. Why not go out and cut the grass, water the plants, read a book or write an email or a blog? Perhaps you could go for a walk and notice the scenery, and observe so many details that in the normal hustle and bustle of daily life you miss.

Try to adopt a really positive attitude towards your lifestyle so that you can substitute healthy calorie-burning activities for unhealthy calorie-consuming ones. The result will be that you'll be fitter and slimmer, and you'll probably enjoy life all the more.

Weight control is about lifestyle more than diet.

RULE 30 Adopt a positive attitude. Exchange calorie-burning activities for calorie-consuming ones.

Modify your whole lifestyle to achieve this end, and you will enjoy your life all the more.

These 30 rules form the basis of how we can control our eating behaviour. In the next chapter we'll summarise them and add a few more weight-loss tips.

Chapter Sixteen

101 WEIGHT-LOSS TIPS

THESE ARE THE TIPS THAT MY clients have found the most useful over the years. They might not all be relevant for you, but I'm sure you will find that many of them can help with your motivation to lose weight and keep slim.

1. Eat sufficient food to satisfy your hunger, but no more.

2. Don't do anything else while you are eating.

3. Always use a knife, fork or spoon for all solid food.

4. When eating out, always choose the smallest portion size available. Faced with larger portions it is all too easy to eat past the point of hunger and therefore consume more calories that contribute to weight gain. If you are still hungry after choosing a smaller meal, you can enjoy eating a small portion of something else that gives you a wider range of flavours to enjoy.

5. Give yourself a time limit for each meal.

6. Put down your knife, fork or spoon between mouthfuls.

7. Cut up your food into as many small pieces as you can.

8. Serve your food on a small plate and spread the food evenly over the plate.

9. Don't keep serving dishes on the table while you eat.

10. Chew your food slowly. Become a gourmet. A gourmet eats slowly, chewing each mouthful of food thoughtfully and lovingly.

11. Swallow each mouthful before you put any more food into your mouth.

12. After finishing your meal get rid of any leftovers immediately.

13. Leave the table as soon as you've finished eating.

14. If you really cannot resist eating chips, choose straight-cut and fatter chips rather than crinkle-cut and thin chips, which hold more fat.

15. Drink a glass of water before a meal. This will partially fill your stomach and will reduce your hunger. Incidentally, hunger is often at least partly due to dehydration.

16. Offer to be the driver for the evening when eating out. This means you'll avoid the calories that come from alcohol.

17. Let others, especially children (if old enough), get their own healthy snacks, such as nuts from the cupboard.

18. Instead of snacking on chocolates or sweets, try eating a handful of unsalted nuts instead. Nuts are filling and, although they are quite high in fat, the fat they contain is good fat that our body needs to stay healthy.

19. Break unhealthy food associations; for example, don't eat while watching TV. Apart from anything else, eating while your attention is elsewhere (such as watching TV) results in the consumption of extra and unneeded calories.

20. If you decide against a planned bicycle ride because it's too windy, think again. Windy conditions make it harder to ride a bike, which means more calories will be burned.

21. If you're out and about, carry a bottle of water with you. It's important to keep well hydrated. Dehydration is often mistaken for hunger – and the last thing you want to do is to fill up with calories when what you need is water.

22. Weekend bingeing is often the undoing of so many people attempting to lose weight. Plan ahead to make sure you have healthy snacks in the house, such as unsalted nuts, low-fat yoghurts, low-calorie soft drinks.

23. When eating out in restaurants, choose lighter options; for example, low-fat dishes, steamed, poached, boiled or baked foods rather than fried foods. But do remember that a lot of pre-packed low-fat foods are high in sugars (see Chapter Ten).

24. Try to reduce the fat, sugar and salt in your diet. Fats and sugars have the most calories – proteins the least. Too much fat can contribute to high cholesterol. Too much salt is linked to health problems, especially high blood pressure.

25. If you enjoy working out in a gym, working out with someone else is great for motivation and keeping you in the groove of regular exercise. This applies to standard workouts and to HIIT.

26. Create a weight-loss challenge with a friend or group of friends. Competing towards a common goal over, say, a six- or 12-week period is a great motivator.

27. Whenever you get the urge to watch TV, but a programme you're really not that interested in, or to be a couch potato, especially at the end of the day, go for a 30-minute walk instead. As well as burning a few calories, this will help you de-stress, clear your mind and relax you before you go to bed.

28. If you have a dessert in a restaurant, why not share it with someone else? That means you can still enjoy the flavour but with far fewer calories. Most restaurants are happy to provide an extra fork and spoon.

29. Use the 'rule of one'. If you simply can't resist a high-calorie treat, allow yourself one small treat a day.

30. Think: *after eight is too late*. This means no snacks after eight o'clock in the evening.

31. Vary your exercise. Doing different kinds of exercise helps to relieve monotony and boredom, and it means you are far more likely to maintain your exercise programme.

32. Before starting a new exercise programme, it's a good idea to gauge your fitness level. A good way to do this is to walk, jog or run for 12 minutes to see what distance you can cover. If you can go 1.6km (1 mile) in 12 minutes or less, you're in fairly good shape. If you're not up to this, start exercising at a comfortable pace and gradually increase your speed as your fitness improves.

33. If you eat meat and poultry, make sure it's lean. This means cutting off any visible fat from red meat and choosing white rather than red poultry meat. This helps to reduce your intake of fat.

34. Remember that portion size matters. Most people find difficulty in losing weight because, although they may eat the right

kinds of food, they eat too much of it. Restaurants often serve portions that are much larger than we need. Try eating just half.

35. Walk during your lunch break. That way, you'll probably eat fewer calories, you'll burn off a few and you'll build up your fitness, but most of all you'll feel more relaxed – and relaxation is so important for weight loss.

36. Park your car further away from the shops and walk. If you use a bus, get off one stop earlier. These are great ways to increase your physical activity.

37. Set realistic weight targets. Don't try to lose weight too quickly. Generally, the quicker the weight loss, the more likely it is for the weight to be piled back on again.

38. Get plenty of sleep. Research shows that lack of sleep increases levels of a hunger hormone and decreases levels of a hormone that makes you feel full.

39. Don't keep tempting foods and snacks in your cupboards. If there are no chocolates, sweets, cakes and so on, you can't eat them – simple!

40. Have some kind of support system in place, such as a slim-buddy. Losing weight is a daily challenge and some days will be more difficult than others. Having someone you can talk to or email can be very helpful.

41. Don't be afraid to snack. People who have small, healthy snacks between meals usually end up consuming fewer calories than those who eat just three meals a day. It's always best not to go into a main meal feeling ravenously hungry.

42. Plan your meals in advance. By planning and, where possible, preparing your meals in advance, those times when you are tempted to grab a quick takeaway and undo all the good you've done with your diet will happen far less often.

43. Create your own dinner deck. This is your 10 favourite quick-and-healthy dinners written on index cards. Each card lists the ingredients and the directions of how to prepare the dish.

44. Keep a food or eating diary. This focuses your mind on what and how much you eat and often results in much less food being eaten. Write down as much information as possible including every single snack. Research shows that people who keep an eating diary lose much more weight than those who don't.

45. When eating out in a restaurant, don't hesitate to ask the waiter or chef to modify your food to ensure that it is healthier, such as grilled rather than fried and smaller portions.

46. Carry a list of foods that you intend to buy when shopping – and stick to it! This will help reduce the temptation to buy chocolates, cakes, biscuits and so on.

47. Don't rely solely on your bathroom scales. Looking at yourself in the mirror and checking how your clothes fit will also provide a useful additional guide to your weight loss.

48. Eat off smaller plates. This is a great way to help control portion sizes.

49. Plateaus happen! Don't fight them. All of us experience periods when weight loss seems to stop for a while. Just accept that, stay motivated and continue with your diet and exercise programme. If the plateau lasts too long, step up your HIIT by an extra minute or two for a few days.

50. Find a photograph of yourself when you were slim and put it in a prominent position to motivate yourself. The fridge is a good place – it should help to reduce temptation.

51. Alternatively, stick a wedding invitation or holiday snaps of places you want to visit on your fridge and use these for motivation to get to the right size in time.

52. When you get a craving to eat something sweet, brush your teeth. This will either put you off eating the food you shouldn't be eating or it may stop you from craving it again in the future.

53. Take up dancing. It's great fun and it burns a lot of calories.

54. Ditch the car or bus or tube, and ride your bike to work. It's a great way to get fit as well as to lose weight. If you live a long way from work, perhaps you can catch a train to work and take your bike and then ride home.

55. Exercise DVDs are a useful way to work out indoors when the weather is really bad, and many of the HIIT routines are suitable for indoors.

56. If you're going to have a treat, work out how much exercise you would need to do to burn off those calories, and tell yourself you'll have the treat only if you do the exercise. Once you realise how many calories a particular treat contains, rather than trying to exercise for a long time (such as a day) to burn it off, you are more likely to forego the treat.

57. Not all hunger is physical – often it is emotional, so try to recognise the difference. Typical features of emotional hunger include: hunger coming on suddenly; hunger involving specific food cravings (such as chocolate); hunger starting in the mouth and the mind, not in the stomach; hunger involving absent-minded eating; hunger that isn't satisfied even when you're full; and – most important of all – hunger that makes you feel guilty.

58. Believe in yourself: believe that you have the power to make the necessary changes in your life.

59. Eat more high-fibre foods. People who have more fibre in their diets tend to have less body fat and a lower body weight.

60. Where possible, eat whole fruits rather than drinking fruit juices. The skins of fruit provide useful fibre. Also, too much fruit juice is not good for tooth enamel and it's a lot of extra sugar, which can upset blood sugar levels.

61. Avoid high-GI foods such as white rice, white bread and well-cooked pasta. A small portion of *al dente* pasta is fine, and choose instead brown rice, long-grain rice and whole-grain products. This helps to avoid blood sugar surges which, in turn, avoid excessive insulin production, therefore helping to avoid fat being deposited in the body. This also helps reduce cravings.

62. Portion size is very important. If you find this difficult, for a while use portion-controlled packaged foods to help you get used to eating smaller portions.

63. Again, if you find controlling portion size difficult, try gradually reducing your serving sizes over time until they reach the ideal size.

64. Don't try to make radical changes to your diet all at once. Instead, make small permanent changes – these are much easier to stick to.

65. Really savour your food. This helps slow down your eating, which allows you to become more conscious of when your stomach is full and may result in your eating less.

66. Never eat while cooking!

67. If you have a starter course for a main meal, choose a light soup or a salad. These are great ways to fill up your stomach with low-calorie, nutritious food.

68. Try to reduce stress in your life and be happy. A feeling of calm and relaxation is important for successful weight loss.

69. Eat a wide range of healthy foods. If you do this, the occasional fast-food meal will be OK.

70. Don't skip breakfast. Choose an egg or whole-grain, high-fibre cereals, such as porridge, with skimmed milk.

71. Learn how to read nutrition labels on packaged food. This will help you make healthy food choices because you can choose the lowest in calories, fat, sugar and salt.

72. Learn to cook new dishes. The more varied your flavours, the more motivated you will be to eat well but healthily. Read cookery magazines or watch TV cookery programmes to get ideas.

73. Use cooking methods that are the least fattening, such as grilling and steaming.

74. If you enjoy alcohol, try to alternate it with low-calorie drinks.

75. Allow yourself to feel good each time you say no to a tempting food.

76. Adopt a reward system that isn't based on food or even weight loss. Instead reward behaviour modifications.

77. Be a role model for your children or partner and set a good example by eating healthily.

78. Encourage your children to eat healthy food that is tasty, well prepared and easy to cook.

79. Shop for food after you've eaten healthy food so that you're less likely to yield to the temptation to buy fast and snack foods.

80. List the shops at which you intend to buy food and don't go into other food shops.

81. Make sure your cupboard is stocked only with healthy foods such as fresh fruit and vegetables, whole-grain cereals and bread, low-fat dairy products, lean meats, poultry and seafood.

82. As much as you can, prepare meals with your children. That way they will learn to enjoy healthy cooking.

83. Don't make children finish their food if they're full. The 'always leave a plate clean' attitude is a leftover from the lean war years and it isn't appropriate for today or good for their health. But of course, in order to avoid waste, give them smaller portions initially with seconds being available.

84. Encourage children to drink water and not to over-indulge in soft drinks and juices, which tend to be loaded with sugar and calories.

85. Teach children good eating habits from a very early age.

86. Encourage children to enjoy sports and be as active as possible.

87. Try not to let your exercise routine slip away during holidays.

88. Never feel obliged to eat just to please others. Eat only what and how much you want. Avoid becoming too hungry. Especially before eating out, it's a good idea to have a very small, healthy snack to take the edge off your hunger so that you don't arrive at a restaurant ravenous.

89. As well as HIIT, think about exercises for strength training for your bones and muscles. This is especially important for women to prevent osteoporosis (thinning of the bones). If you have the time, stretching for flexibility of ligaments and tendons is also good.

90. Don't become over-enthusiastic about your weight-loss target. Remember that being too thin can be hazardous to your health. Aim for a BMI of between 18.5 and 25 (see pages 15–18).

91. If you feel that your weight-loss target is too far away to take on board, remember that even a 10 per cent weight loss brings enormous health benefits.

92. Don't try to cut out dietary fat completely. Some fat is important for our health. Fat is necessary for building body tissue and aiding the absorption of some vitamins and minerals.

93. Rather than buying larger clothes, if you've put on weight, diet and exercise until your clothes fit comfortably again.

94. Keep fruit in a bowl. Fruit provides a healthy snack. Within reason, you can eat as much as you like of fruit from temperate climates, such as apples and pears, but you should limit your consumption of fruit from exotic climates, such as mangos, as they contain a lot of sugar.

95. If you feel stressed or bored, go for a walk or do some other form of exercise rather than turning to food. Quite apart from preventing the consumption of unnecessary calories, exercise is a great way to relieve stress or boredom.

96. Sushi has become a very popular lunchtime choice – it can be low in calories and can be very healthy, if you choose wisely; for example, choose brown rice if it's available, although unfortunately it often isn't. If you're eating maki, limit yourself to two rolls. Spicy tuna rolls usually have added mayonnaise, so eat no more than one. The healthiest rolls are seafood and veggie ones. Avoid tempura, which, being battered and deep-fried, is full of fat and calories.

97. Low-fat Greek yoghurt is the dieter's friend. It's high in protein and this means you'll feel fuller for longer after eating it. And it's very versatile. You can mix it with fresh fruit and/or with artificial sweetener, for example.

98. Avoid foods with more than 10 per cent fat; that is, more than 10g fat per 100g (3½oz) food.

99. If you slip up by over-indulging, don't give up. Be like a champion skater: if you fall, pick yourself up and carry on even better than you did before.

100. If you're fond of coffee, especially coffee with milk, try to replace some of your coffee drinks with herbal teas, which require no milk and are very soothing. There are lots of different flavours, so you can enjoy a great variety.

101. Swap calorie-consuming activities for calorie-burning ones.

All of the above should help you to adopt a positive attitude, which will help you to modify your whole lifestyle towards achieving your goal. And you'll enjoy your life all the more.

Part Five

FOOD – THE BASICS FOR HEALTHY EATING AND WEIGHT LOSS

Chapter Seventeen

THE HEALTHY STORE-CUPBOARD AND COOKING TIPS

H AVING A STORE-CUPBOARD of healthy foods is the biggest step towards achieving your weight loss and staying there.

DAIRY PRODUCTS

There is a wide range of dairy products that are good for my approach to losing weight without really dieting, because the sugar they contain, which is lactose, is absorbed quite slowly into the bloodstream. Especially good for weight control are the low-fat versions (but remember to check that they don't contain sugar or carbohydrate fillers in place of the fat – see page 123). Find a place for:

► Milk: skimmed or semi-skimmed.

► Yoghurt: plain or flavoured low-fat or non-fat.

▶ Cheese: low- or non-fat versions – less than 5g fat per 25g (1oz) – of cottage cheese, ricotta cheese, feta cheese, cream cheese, mozzarella cheese, Swiss cheeses, Cheddar cheese, Parmesan cheese for sprinkling on other foods. If you dislike low-fat hard cheeses, choose stronger cheeses, such as a mature Cheddar, and eat them in *very small* amounts.

▶ Low-fat ice creams and sorbets.

▶ Spreads: light butter or light margarine, in small amounts (see page 145). Avoid hydrogenated kinds.

OILS, MAYONNAISE AND SALAD DRESSINGS

▶ Oils: rapeseed, soya oil, walnut oil, non-stick vegetable oil cooking spray are good used in very small quantities for cooking. Olive oil, preferably extra virgin olive oil, is best for salads.

▶ Mayonnaise: light or non-fat.

▶ Salad dressings: low-fat or non-fat.

EGGS

Far from being the villains they were once believed to be, eggs contain no saturated fat and raise our good blood cholesterol (HDL) more than the bad (LDL). They also contain nutrients that may help lower the risk of heart disease, including protein, vitamins B_{12}, D and E, riboflavin and folate. Up to seven egg yolks a week is fine, but if you have diabetes you should probably limit yourself to no more than two or three eggs a week, as the Nurses' Health Study found that for diabetics an egg a day might increase the risk of heart disease.[6] Also, if you have difficulty controlling your blood cholesterol or if you have heart disease or diabetes, you need to be a little careful about eating egg yolks and eat no more than one a day. For everyone, egg whites are unlimited. If you can find them, choose omega-3-enriched eggs.

MEAT, POULTRY AND FISH

► Lean cuts of all meats. Trim off visible fat.

► Back bacon.

► Any fresh or frozen fish or shellfish, but try especially to include oily fish such as salmon and mackerel.

► Any tinned fish in water or brine, such as tuna. Avoid fish tinned in oil.

BREADS

Avoid breads, bagels, burger buns and muffins made from finely ground flour. The best breads to eat are:

► 100 per cent stoneground wholemeal bread – one thin slice.

► Pumpernickel bread – one slice.

► Multigrain breads – one thin slice.

► Rye bread – one thin slice.

► Sourdough bread, which has a moderately low GI because of its acidity – one thin slice.

▶ Wholemeal pitta bread – one small pitta bread.

▶ Wholemeal flour tortillas – one small tortilla.

PASTA AND NOODLES

All pastas are fine provided you cook them *al dente* and you eat small portions, 50g (1¾oz) raw weight only. Stock up on:

▶ Varieties of pasta, especially wholegrain.

▶ Noodles.

RICE AND OTHER GRAINS

Avoid sticky white rice. Instead choose:

▶ Long-grain rice, long-grain brown rice, basmati rice, Uncle Ben's rice (this rice has been steamed prior to milling).

▶ Buckwheat – used, for example, in kasha.

▶ Barley – used in casseroles, pilaffs and soups.

▶ Bulgur wheat (cracked wheat) – used in many dishes including casseroles and pilaffs.

▶ Couscous.

▶ Polenta (cornmeal).

PULSES

These can be bought dried or canned and ready to use. Drain and rinse before adding to your recipe. Pulses include:

▶ Black beans.

▶ Cannellini beans.

▶ Chickpeas (such as in hummus).

▶ Haricot beans.

▶ Kidney beans.

▶ Lentils.

FLOURS

▶ Whole-grain flours (also known as wholewheat or wholemeal).

▶ Wheatgerm flour.

BREAKFAST CEREALS

▶ Shredded Wheat and Weetabix.

▶ Porridge made with rolled oats (not instant porridge).

THE CHANGING WORLD OF BREAKFAST

In recent years there has been a major change in healthy recommendations for breakfast cereals. In 2012 the independent consumer watchdog Which? published an analysis of the nutritional value of breakfast cereals. It compared the sugar, salt and fat content of 50 cereals, based on the manufacturers' information. It found that overall, 32 out of the 50 were high in sugar, and that 12 out of the 14 cereals aimed at children had excessive levels of added sugar. But there was some good news: most cereals have reduced their salt levels over the last few years. The official traffic-light labelling system defines excessive levels of sugar as more than 12.5 per cent sugar (12.5g per 100g/3½oz). In only two of these cereals this was due to the fruit they contained. For the rest it was due to added sugar. The report said that Nestlé Shredded Wheat was the healthiest cereal with low levels of sugar, fat and salt. The only other cereals that were low in sugar were Quaker Oat So Simple Original and Weetabix. The downside with Quaker Oat So Simple is that it contained medium fat levels (8.5g per 100g/3½oz), whereas Weetabix contained medium salt levels (0.65g per 100g/3½oz). But before you discard the idea of breakfast cereals, it's worth bearing in mind that, compared with a full English breakfast, the average cereal is still probably a better option. Further, most breakfast cereals are fortified with vitamins and minerals. But of course there many other healthy breakfast options, such as scrambled eggs on wholemeal toast, porridge made with rolled oats and skimmed milk, or a raw vegetable muesli – carrot, apple and cinnamon muesli (available online from www.primroseskitchen.com).

TINNED FOODS

► Tuna in brine.

► Salmon or sardines in water.

► Corn.

► Fruits in natural juices.

► Pulses (see page 189).

CONDIMENTS AND HERBS

All condiments and herbs are OK, but use tomato ketchup in moderation. Depending on the style of food you like to cook, stock up with:

► Dried herbs, such as mixed herbs, thyme, oregano, bay leaves (parsley and leaf coriander are best used fresh) – all are good in Mediterranean cooking.

► Ground spices, such as cumin, coriander, ginger, turmeric, Chinese five-spice powder – used in Middle Eastern and Asian dishes.

► Cajun seasoning, dried chilli flakes.

FRUIT AND VEGETABLES

Most fruit and vegetables are OK, but limit quantities of potatoes (other than small new and sweet potatoes), parsnips, carrots (other than small portions) and watermelon. Eat at least five portions of vegetables and fruit a day. Dried apricots are fine, because they have a low GI compared to other dried fruits. (Serve four dried apricots as a dessert or have one as a snack.) Stock up with:

▶ Green leafy vegetables: broccoli, kale, cabbage, lettuce, mixed salad leaves.

▶ Tomatoes, aubergines, peppers, chillies.

▶ Courgettes, marrows.

▶ Fresh or frozen peas, broad beans, green beans.

▶ Butternut squash.

▶ Asparagus.

NUTS AND SEEDS

▶ Almonds, pecan nuts, pine nuts, walnuts, cashew nuts, hazelnuts.

▶ Peanuts and peanut butter (in small amounts – remember, it is quite calorific). Choose butters without palm oil as these are usually partially hydrogenated.

▶ Flaxseeds, sesame seeds, sunflower seeds, pumpkin seeds.

COOKING TIPS FOR CUTTING CALORIES OR THE GI

▶ **Pastas** Cook *al dente*. Try to include vegetables in pasta recipes.

▶ **Breaded coatings** Use Special K rather than breadcrumbs.

▶ **Meat** Use lean cuts and trim off visible fat. Cooking methods: grill, stir-fry, oven-fry (lightly coat in oil and bake instead of fry – as in home-made oven chips), bake.

▶ **Omelettes** Use lean meats, low-fat cheeses and lots of vegetables.

▶ **Casseroles** Use basmati, long-grain brown, parboiled (as in Uncle Ben's rice) or wild rice, or bulgur wheat instead of regular long-grain white rice. Use lower-fat cheeses or soured cream. Include plenty of pulses and vegetables. Use as little oil, butter or margarine as possible.

▶ **Soups** Use basmati, long-grain brown, parboiled (as in Uncle Ben's rice) or wild rice or barley instead of regular long-grain white rice. Include plenty of pulses, vegetables and pasta. Use skimmed or semi-skimmed milk rather than whole milk. Thicken with puréed vegetables rather than cream.

▶ **Burgers and meatballs** Use extra-lean meat. Add cooked lentils, pulses, rolled oats, oat bran or bulgur wheat instead of white rice or breadcrumbs. Include lots of chopped vegetables.

▶ **Stuffings** Use low-GI breads and lots of chopped vegetables.

▶ **Sauces** Use skimmed or semi-skimmed milk rather than whole milk. Use as little butter or margarine as possible.

▶ **Marinades** Use more fruit juices with less sugar for sweetness.

▶ **Salads** Use low-fat mayonnaise and dressings or soured cream. Use lean meats and lower-fat cheeses.

▶ **Pancakes and Yorkshire pudding batter** Use oat bran, wheat bran, wheatgerm or ground flaxseed instead of some of the flour. Serve pancakes with low-sugar fruit sauce or apple sauce or fruit (fresh or tinned in natural juice).

▶ **Custards and puddings** Use skimmed or semi-skimmed milk rather than whole milk. Use vanilla, cinnamon or nutmeg instead of some, or all, of the sugar.

▶ **Sandwiches** Use low-GI breads (see page 99) and lots of vegetables.

Chapter Eighteen

INTRODUCTION TO THE RECIPES

IT'S NOW TIME TO GET DOWN to business and focus on the diet element of the 12-Minute Weight-Loss Plan. This diet is very different from other popular diets such as low-fat and high-protein/low-carb diets. The point of it is that to lose weight you need to watch not only fats but carbs as well. But please note: you are *watching* carbs, not *cutting them out completely*! It's the quality of the carbs that counts. The wrong carbs will make your body pump out lots of insulin, which pushes fat into your body's cells and stops that fat from getting out again. The right carbs, on the other hand, encourage your body to burn off fat and satisfy your hunger for much longer so that you end up eating less.

This diet is about eating the right foods, which means a healthy balance of proteins, fats and the right carbs, and preparing or cooking that food in a way that doesn't encourage your body to lay down fat. If you follow the advice and follow the exercise plan, you *will* lose weight. Equally importantly, you will enjoy good, tasty food and you won't be hungry. And the icing on the cake – if you'll forgive an inappropriate metaphor in a book on diet – is that you'll reap health benefits, so you will have less likelihood of developing coronary heart disease or diabetes.

A TWO-PHASE APPROACH

Like all good (and bad) slimming books, there are two phases to this eating programme: Orientation (Phase 1) and Continuation (Phase 2). Why? Simply because most of us who have quite a bit of weight to shed need a kick-start. It's all about motivation.

The other reason for an Orientation Phase is that it's a useful phase to return to in future if you've been a bit 'naughty' and put on some weight again – perhaps because of Christmas or a holiday.

Orientation lasts for two weeks. As you'd expect, there are tighter guidelines regarding what you can and can't eat. Then, after two weeks, you go on to Continuation. This lasts for the rest of your life. But remember, you will enjoy Continuation. (You'll enjoy Orientation too, but Continuation will be that much more fun.) You're going to be eating lots of wonderful, tasty foods and you won't be feeling hungry. Enjoy!

For each phase you will find two weeks of suggested menus for every meal. I strongly suggest that in Orientation, at least, you stick as closely as you can to those suggestions. But if you find there is a food that you really don't like, then by all means replace that meal suggestion with another. It is important that you enjoy the diet from the very start. The menus for Orientation follow in the next chapter.

WELCOME TO ORIENTATION

As you will have come to expect by now, you'll find lots of suggestions for a healthy, nutritious, delicious and well-balanced diet. You will find too that there are carbs, but not as many as you will be able to have once you go on to Continuation. The list of foods for Orientation is on the pages that follow.

Before we begin, have a quick look at the foods you can eat and those you should avoid. You will find these on the next couple of pages.

PHASE 1, ORIENTATION – FOODS TO INCLUDE AND FOODS TO AVOID

	Foods to include	Foods to avoid
Alcohol		All alcohol
Breads	Wheat tortillas	All breads
Cereals		All cereals
Cheese	Low-fat cottage cheese Any low-fat version of other cheeses Feta Mozzarella Parmesan Ricotta	Medium- and high-fat cheeses, such as Brie, Edam and Stilton
Cooking oil	Rapeseed oil Olive oil	
Dairy	Skimmed milk Soya milk Low-fat yoghurts, plain and fruit	Whole or semi-skimmed milk Yoghurt, non low-fatIce cream
Eggs	Yolks: as you like, but follow any medical advice you may have been given Whites: unlimited	
Pulses	Hummus	

▶

	Foods to include	**Foods to avoid**
Fruit	Dried apricots Cherries Grapefruit – 3 times a day! Prunes	All fruits except in left-hand column
Fruit juices	Tomato juice	All juices except in left-hand column
Lentils and pulses	Butter beans Chickpeas Kidney beans Lentils Soya beans (also available frozen)	
Meat	Lean cuts with no visible fat of: Beef liver Pork, including ham and bacon Veal	All fatty meats and visible fat
Nuts	All, but there are daily limits; choose one from the list per day: Brazil nuts 10 Cashew nuts 15 Peanuts 20 Peanut butter – 15g (½oz)/1 tbsp Pistachio nuts 30 Walnuts 15	
Pasta		All pasta
Poultry	White meat without skin: Chicken breast Turkey breast	Poultry red meat: Chicken wings and legs Turkey wings and legs Chicken liver Duck Goose
Rice		All rice
Seafood	All fish and shellfish	
Spices and sauces	All non-sugared sauces and spices (check the labels) Horseradish sauce Pepper sauce	

▶

	Foods to include	Foods to avoid
Vegetables	All green vegetables Artichoke Aubergine Cauliflower Lemon juice, lime juice Mushrooms Onions Peppers Radishes Tomatoes	All except in left-hand column
Miscellaneous	Horseradish sauce Pepper Salt – as little as possible Soy sauce Worcestershire sauce	Tomato ketchup
Drinks	Tea* Coffee* (2 cups a day) Decaffeinated coffee (unlimited) Low-calorie soft drinks (limit 2 drinks a day unless caffeine-free)	Excess coffee Non-low-calorie soft drinks Excess low-calorie soft drinks unless caffeine-free

* Tea and coffee to be drunk preferably black or with a dash of skimmed milk; no sugar (but artificial sweetener allowed).

TIME TO GET READY FOR THE ORIENTATION PHASE

The recipes are generally simple and quick. This is to help keep you out of the kitchen as much as possible. In particular, the evening meal has the minimum of preparation time and washing up. The number of vegetables is kept to a minimum – and generally includes just one! I encourage you to drink a lot of water. There are many reasons for this, but the two most important ones are:

1. Lack of water causes dehydration even if you don't feel thirsty. And dehydration makes you tired and lethargic, and less enthusiastic about everything – including your diet!

2. Water fills your stomach up and helps you to feel satisfied with less food.

Grapefruit – that something extra

You may have heard of the Grapefruit Diet. It's been around for a long time – since the 1930s in fact. And various incarnations of this diet seem to have worked to some extent. The diet involves starting off each meal with half a grapefruit and is usually combined with a very low-calorie diet as well. But the problem has always been that the diet has been too restrictive for people to follow indefinitely. And, until recently, no one has understood why grapefruit could help weight loss.

In 2006 a paper was published which reported the results of a 12-week study carried out on 100 obese people in the US. One group ate half a grapefruit three times a day before each meal. Another drank a glass of grapefruit juice before every meal. A third did not include grapefruit in their meals. The group eating grapefruit without otherwise changing their diet lost an average of 3.6 pounds (1.6kg), some shedding as much as 10 pounds (4.5kg). The group drinking grapefruit juice, again without otherwise changing their diet, lost an average of 3.3 pounds (1.5kg). The control group, who consumed no grapefruit, lost an average of only ½ pound (225g).[7]

By measuring blood glucose levels, the researchers believed that the weight loss was probably linked to lowered levels of insulin. Insulin is used to metabolise sugar, as we have seen. The more efficiently sugar is metabolised, the less likely it is to be stored as fat in the body. Also, lowering insulin levels makes you feel less hungry. High levels of insulin, on the other hand, cause hunger and stimulate the liver to manufacture fat, which increases body weight and also causes coronary heart disease.

The inclusion of grapefruit at each meal helps weight loss, reduces the risk of coronary heart disease and lowers the risk of developing type-2 diabetes. (**NOTE:** It's important, however, to see the warning about grapefruit interactions with certain medications in Appendix 2.)

If you really don't like grapefruit, you can leave it out. It's completely optional.

Otherwise, during the Orientation Phase, you eat half a grapefruit before each of your three main meals each day. You can, of course, carry this on into the Continuation Phase. Indeed, if you still have weight to lose after Orientation it is important that you *do* continue with grapefruit. Again, remember though: the grapefruit is optional.

In the next chapter you will find menus for each of the 14 days of the Orientation Phase.

Most importantly – enjoy! Enjoy reading, enjoy losing weight – and enjoy your food.

Chapter Nineteen

THE ORIENTATION PHASE
DAILY MENUS

N THE MENUS THAT FOLLOW you will find an exact daily menu. Recipes are provided for meals marked with *.

DAY 1

BREAKFAST
A glass of water

Optional: half a grapefruit (with optional artificial sweetener)

An egg poached in water with a splash of vinegar and with
2 rashers of grilled lean back bacon

Tea or decaffeinated coffee with optional skimmed milk
and sweetener, but no sugar

MORNING SNACK
A glass of water

5 Brazil nuts, *or* 25g (1oz) flaxseeds or sesame seeds. (If you wish,
use seeds as alternatives to nuts throughout the menus.)

LUNCH
A glass of water

Optional: half a grapefruit (with optional artificial sweetener)

4 tbsp cottage cheese, sprinkled with 2 chopped dried apricots

AFTERNOON SNACK
A glass of water

A bowl of cherries or berries (fresh or thawed frozen)

DINNER
A glass of water

Optional: half a grapefruit (with optional artificial sweetener)

Herbed Mustardy Chicken* served with green vegetables

Ricotta Cheese Dessert* *or* plain or fruit low-fat yoghurt,
or a small bowl of cherries or berries (fresh or thawed frozen),
or 4 dried apricots, *or* either the yoghurt or fruit
with sugar-free jelly

Tea or decaffeinated coffee with optional skimmed milk
and sweetener, but no sugar

DAY 2

BREAKFAST
A glass of water

Optional: half a grapefruit (with optional artificial sweetener)

Low-fat fruit yoghurt

Tea or decaffeinated coffee with optional skimmed milk and
sweetener, but no sugar

MORNING SNACK
A glass of water

Celery stick stuffed with any low-fat cheese, such as cottage
cheese, Laughing Cow light cheese

LUNCH
A glass of water

Optional: half a grapefruit (with optional artificial sweetener)

Mixed green salad – as much as you want

AFTERNOON SNACK
A glass of water

8 cashew nuts

DINNER
A glass of water

Optional: half a grapefruit (with optional artificial sweetener)

A glass of tomato juice

Pork Medallions with Apricots* served with green vegetables

Ricotta Cheese Dessert*, *or* plain or fruit low-fat yoghurt,
or a small bowl of cherries or berries (fresh or thawed frozen),
or 4 dried apricots, *or* either the yoghurt or fruit with
sugar-free jelly

Tea or decaffeinated coffee with optional skimmed milk
and sweetener, but no sugar

DAY 3

BREAKFAST
A glass of water

Optional: half a grapefruit (with optional artificial sweetener)

2-egg omelette with 2 rashers of grilled lean back bacon

Tea or decaffeinated coffee with optional skimmed milk
and sweetener, but no sugar

MORNING SNACK
A glass of water

10 unsalted peanuts

LUNCH
A glass of water

Optional: half a grapefruit (with optional artificial sweetener)

75g (2¾oz) lean diced ham

Mixed green salad – as much as you want

AFTERNOON SNACK
A glass of water

Celery stick with hummus

DINNER
A glass of water

Optional: half a grapefruit (with optional artificial sweetener)

A glass of tomato juice

Grilled Cod with Broccoli*

Ricotta Cheese Dessert*, or plain or fruit low-fat yoghurt,
or a small bowl of cherries or berries (fresh or thawed frozen),
or 4 dried apricots, or either the yoghurt or fruit with
sugar-free jelly

Tea or decaffeinated coffee with optional skimmed milk
and sweetener, but no sugar

DAY 4

BREAKFAST
A glass of water

Optional: half a grapefruit (with optional artificial sweetener)

Low-fat fruit yoghurt

Tea or decaffeinated coffee with optional skimmed milk
and sweetener, but no sugar

MORNING SNACK
A glass of water

Celery stick stuffed with any low-fat cheese, such as
cottage cheese, Laughing Cow light cheese

LUNCH
A glass of water

Optional: half a grapefruit (with optional artificial sweetener)

100g (3½oz) white tuna – in brine or water, only

Mixed green salad – as much as you want

AFTERNOON SNACK
A glass of water

8 walnuts

DINNER
A glass of water

Optional: half a grapefruit (with optional artificial sweetener)

A glass of tomato juice

Beef and Vegetable Stir-fry*

Ricotta Cheese Dessert*, or plain or fruit low-fat yoghurt, or a
small bowl of cherries or berries (fresh or thawed frozen), or 4
dried apricots, or either the yoghurt or fruit with sugar-free jelly

Tea or decaffeinated coffee with optional skimmed milk
and sweetener, but no sugar

DAY 5

BREAKFAST
A glass of water

Optional: half a grapefruit (with optional artificial sweetener)

Low-fat plain yoghurt

Tea or decaffeinated coffee with optional skimmed milk
and sweetener, but no sugar

MORNING SNACK
A glass of water

A bowl of cherries or berries (fresh or thawed frozen)

LUNCH
A glass of water

Optional: half a grapefruit (with optional artificial sweetener)

100g (3½oz) grilled chicken breast with skin and fat removed

Mixed green salad – as much as you want

AFTERNOON SNACK
A glass of water

4 dried apricots

DINNER
A glass of water

Optional: half a grapefruit (with optional artificial sweetener)

A glass of tomato juice

Creamy Veal Escalope* with French beans

Ricotta Cheese Dessert*, *or* plain or fruit low-fat yoghurt, *or* a
small bowl of cherries or berries (fresh or thawed frozen), *or* 4
dried apricots, *or* either the yoghurt or fruit with sugar-free jelly

Tea or decaffeinated coffee with optional skimmed milk
and sweetener, but no sugar

DAY 6

BREAKFAST
A glass of water

Optional: half a grapefruit (with optional artificial sweetener)

2 scrambled eggs with 2 rashers of grilled lean back bacon

Tea or decaffeinated coffee with optional skimmed milk
and sweetener, but no sugar

MORNING SNACK
A glass of water

Celery stick stuffed with any low-fat cheese, such as cottage
cheese, Laughing Cow light cheese

LUNCH
A glass of water

Optional: half a grapefruit (with optional artificial sweetener)

Gazpacho*

Low-fat fruit yoghurt

AFTERNOON SNACK
A glass of water

8 cashew nuts

DINNER
A glass of water

Optional: half a grapefruit (with optional artificial sweetener)

A glass of tomato juice

Fillet of Beef with Asparagus* accompanied by a small bowl of
green salad

Ricotta Cheese Dessert*, or plain or fruit low-fat yoghurt, or a
small bowl of cherries or berries (fresh or thawed frozen), or 4
dried apricots, or either the yoghurt or fruit with sugar-free jelly

Tea or decaffeinated coffee with optional skimmed milk
and sweetener, but no sugar

DAY 7

BREAKFAST
A glass of water
Optional: half a grapefruit (with optional artificial sweetener)
Low-fat fruit yoghurt
Tea or decaffeinated coffee with optional skimmed milk
and sweetener, but no sugar

MORNING SNACK
A glass of water
15 pistachio nuts

LUNCH
A glass of water
4 tbsp cottage cheese
Mixed green salad – as much as you want

AFTERNOON SNACK
A glass of water
Celery stick with hummus

DINNER
A glass of water
Optional: half a grapefruit (with optional artificial sweetener)
A glass of tomato juice
Turkey Curry* with green beans
Ricotta Cheese Dessert*, *or* plain or fruit low-fat yoghurt, *or* a
small bowl of cherries or berries (fresh or thawed frozen), *or* 4
dried apricots, *or* either the yoghurt or fruit with sugar-free jelly
Tea or decaffeinated coffee with optional skimmed milk
and sweetener, but no sugar

DAY 8

BREAKFAST
A glass of water

Optional: half a grapefruit (with optional artificial sweetener)

2-egg omelette with 2 rashers of grilled lean back bacon

Tea or decaffeinated coffee with optional skimmed milk
and sweetener, but no sugar

MORNING SNACK
A glass of water

Celery stick stuffed with any low-fat cheese, such as cottage
cheese, Laughing Cow light cheese

LUNCH
A glass of water

Optional: half a grapefruit (with optional artificial sweetener)

100g (3½oz) lean diced ham

Mixed green salad – as much as you want

AFTERNOON SNACK
A glass of water

8 walnuts

DINNER
A glass of water

Optional: half a grapefruit (with optional artificial sweetener)

A glass of tomato juice

Grilled Salmon with Spinach*

Ricotta Cheese Dessert*, *or* plain or fruit low-fat yoghurt, *or* a
small bowl of cherries or berries (fresh or thawed frozen), *or* 4
dried apricots, *or* either the yoghurt or fruit with sugar-free jelly

Tea or decaffeinated coffee with optional skimmed milk
and sweetener, but no sugar

DAY 9

BREAKFAST
A glass of water

Optional: half a grapefruit (with optional artificial sweetener)

Low-fat fruit yoghurt

Tea or decaffeinated coffee with optional skimmed milk
and sweetener, but no sugar

MORNING SNACK
A glass of water

15 pistachio nuts

LUNCH
A glass of water

Optional: half a grapefruit (with optional artificial sweetener)

120g (4¼oz) grilled turkey breast

Mixed green salad – as much as you can manage

AFTERNOON SNACK
A glass of water

A bowl of cherries or berries (fresh or thawed frozen)

DINNER
A glass of water

Optional: half a grapefruit (with optional artificial sweetener)

A glass of tomato juice

Mexican Beef Stir-fry* accompanied by a mixed green salad

Ricotta Cheese Dessert*, or plain or fruit low-fat yoghurt, or a
small bowl of cherries or berries (fresh or thawed frozen), or 4
dried apricots, or either the yoghurt or fruit with sugar-free jelly

Tea or decaffeinated coffee with optional skimmed milk
and sweetener, but no sugar

DAY 10

BREAKFAST
A glass of water

Optional: half a grapefruit (with optional artificial sweetener)

2 scrambled eggs with 2 rashers of grilled lean back bacon

Tea or decaffeinated coffee with optional skimmed milk
and sweetener, but no sugar

MORNING SNACK
A glass of water

Celery stick stuffed with any low-fat cheese, such as cottage
cheese, Laughing Cow light cheese

LUNCH
A glass of water

Optional: half a grapefruit (with optional artificial sweetener)

100g (3½oz) tuna – in brine or water only

Mixed green salad – as much as you can manage

AFTERNOON SNACK
A glass of water

5 Brazil nuts

DINNER
A glass of water

Optional: half a grapefruit (with optional artificial sweetener)

A glass of tomato juice

Herbed Plaice with Broccoli*

Ricotta Cheese Dessert*, *or* plain or fruit low-fat yoghurt, *or* a
small bowl of cherries or berries (fresh or thawed frozen), *or* 4
dried apricots, *or* either the yoghurt or fruit with sugar-free jelly

Tea or decaffeinated coffee with optional skimmed milk
and sweetener, but no sugar

DAY 11

BREAKFAST
A glass of water

Optional: half a grapefruit (with optional artificial sweetener)

2 eggs, poached in water, with a dash of vinegar, with 2 rashers of grilled lean back bacon

Tea or decaffeinated coffee with optional skimmed milk and sweetener, but no sugar

MORNING SNACK
A glass of water

4 dried apricots

LUNCH
A glass of water

Optional: half a grapefruit (with optional artificial sweetener)

Tomato soup*

Low-fat fruit yoghurt

AFTERNOON SNACK
A glass of water

8 cashew nuts

DINNER
A glass of water

Optional: half a grapefruit (with optional artificial sweetener)

A glass of tomato juice

Peanut Chicken* accompanied by greens

Ricotta Cheese Dessert*, *or* plain or fruit low-fat yoghurt, *or* a small bowl of cherries or berries (fresh or thawed frozen), *or* 4 dried apricots, *or* either the yoghurt or fruit with sugar-free jelly

Tea or decaffeinated coffee with optional skimmed milk and sweetener, but no sugar

DAY 12

BREAKFAST
A glass of water

Optional: half a grapefruit (with optional artificial sweetener)

Low-fat fruit yoghurt

Tea or decaffeinated coffee with optional skimmed milk
and sweetener, but no sugar

MORNING SNACK
A glass of water

Celery stick stuffed with any low-fat cheese, such as cottage
cheese, Laughing Cow light cheese

LUNCH
A glass of water

Optional: half a grapefruit (with optional artificial sweetener)

75g (2¾oz) lean diced ham

Mixed green salad – as much as you can manage

AFTERNOON SNACK
A glass of water

10 unsalted peanuts

DINNER
A glass of water

Optional: half a grapefruit (with optional artificial sweetener)

A glass of tomato juice

Spiced Turkey with Courgettes*

Ricotta Cheese Dessert*, *or* plain or fruit low-fat yoghurt, *or* a
small bowl of cherries or berries (fresh or thawed frozen), *or* 4
dried apricots, *or* either the yoghurt or fruit with sugar-free jelly

Tea or decaffeinated coffee with optional skimmed milk
and sweetener, but no sugar

DAY 13

BREAKFAST
A glass of water

Optional: half a grapefruit (with optional artificial sweetener)

2 scrambled eggs with 2 rashers of grilled lean back bacon

Tea or decaffeinated coffee with optional skimmed milk
and sweetener, but no sugar

MORNING SNACK
A glass of water

15 pistachio nuts

LUNCH
A glass of water

Optional: half a grapefruit (with optional artificial sweetener)

120g (4¼oz) grilled turkey breast

Mixed green salad – as much as you can manage

AFTERNOON SNACK
A glass of water

A bowl of cherries or berries (fresh or thawed frozen)

DINNER
A glass of water

Optional: half a grapefruit (with optional artificial sweetener)

A glass of tomato juice

Prawns with Rocket Dressing and Asparagus*

Ricotta Cheese Dessert*, or plain or fruit low-fat yoghurt, or a
small bowl of cherries or berries (fresh or thawed frozen), or 4
dried apricots, or either the yoghurt or fruit with sugar-free jelly

Tea or decaffeinated coffee with optional skimmed milk
and sweetener, but no sugar

DAY 14

BREAKFAST
A glass of water

Optional: half a grapefruit (with optional artificial sweetener)

Low-fat plain yoghurt

Tea or decaffeinated coffee with optional skimmed milk
and sweetener, but no sugar

MORNING SNACK
A glass of water

Celery stick stuffed with any low-fat cheese, such as cottage
cheese, Laughing Cow light cheese

LUNCH
A glass of water

Optional: half a grapefruit (with optional artificial sweetener)

Orientation Phase Lentil Soup*

Low-fat fruit yoghurt

AFTERNOON SNACK
A glass of water

8 walnuts

DINNER
A glass of water

Optional: half a grapefruit (with optional artificial sweetener)

A glass of tomato juice

Curried Pork Medallions* accompanied by French beans

Ricotta Cheese Dessert*, *or* plain or fruit low-fat yoghurt, *or* a
small bowl of cherries or berries (fresh or thawed frozen), *or* 4
dried apricots, *or* either the yoghurt or fruit with sugar-free jelly

Tea or decaffeinated coffee with optional skimmed milk
and sweetener, but no sugar

Chapter Twenty

RECIPES FOR THE ORIENTATION PHASE

THE RECIPES ARE IN THE order of the daily menus. The dessert for this phase is on page 228.

Herbed Mustardy Chicken

SERVES 4

4 tsp English mustard
4 tbsp chopped fresh herbs, such as parsley, oregano,
   rosemary, plus extra to garnish
4 skinless chicken breasts, about 125g (4½oz) each
a pinch of salt
freshly ground black pepper

Put the mustard, herbs and 1 tsp water in a bowl and combine into a paste, then use this to smother both sides of the chicken breasts. Season on both sides with salt and pepper.

Preheat the grill to low. Put the chicken in a grill pan or baking tray and grill for 15–20 minutes until cooked though and the juices run clear. Garnish with herbs.

Pork Medallions with Apricots

SERVES 4

6 dried apricots, soaked overnight and drained
rapeseed oil, for frying
650g (1lb 7oz) pork fillet (tenderloin), cut into medallions
2cm (¾in) thick
a pinch of salt
freshly ground black pepper

Put the apricots in a blender and process to make a purée. Add a smear of oil to a non-stick frying pan and add the pork. Cook over a medium heat for 5 minutes on each side or until cooked through.

Heat the apricot purée gently in a small pan. Season and serve with the pork.

Grilled Cod with Broccoli

SERVES 4

1 tbsp olive oil
1 tsp lemon juice
1 tbsp chopped fresh parsley
4 portions cod fillet, about 680g (1½lb) total weight
a pinch of salt
freshly ground black pepper
lightly steamed broccoli, to serve

Put the olive oil in a bowl and add the lemon juice, parsley and salt and pepper. Mix into a paste and use to spread over the top of each cod fillet. Preheat the grill to medium.

Put the cod in a grill pan or baking tray and grill for 10–15 minutes until cooked through and the fish flakes easily with a knife. Do not over-cook. Serve with the broccoli.

Beef and Vegetable Stir-fry

SERVES 4

> 1 tbsp rapeseed oil
> 450g (1lb) rump steak, cut into thin slices
> green vegetables of your choice, as much as you can manage,
>   cut into even-sized pieces
> soy sauce, to taste

Heat the oil in a wok or large pan over a medium-high heat and stir-fry the beef slices until seared. Add the vegetables and soy sauce, then stir-fry until tender but still crisp – do not over-cook. Add a little water, if needed.

Creamy Veal Escalope

SERVES 4

> ½ tsp olive oil
> ½ tsp rapeseed oil
> 4 veal escalopes, about 450g (1lb) total weight
> 4 slices of low-fat cheese
> 1 tsp Marsala wine (no more – this is the Orientation Phase!)
> a pinch of dried sage
> a pinch of salt

freshly ground black pepper
lightly steamed French beans, to serve (as much as you can
   manage)

Heat the oils in a non-stick frying pan over a medium heat. Season the veal and fry it for 1–2 minutes on each side until golden and tender and almost cooked.

Add the wine and sage to the pan and cook for 1 minute to cook off the alcohol. Put a slice of cheese on top of each escalope and serve with the French beans.

Gazpacho

SERVES 4

450g (1lb) tomatoes
85ml (3fl oz) beef stock
½ green or red pepper, deseeded and roughly chopped
1 tbsp wine vinegar
1 courgette, roughly chopped
1 cucumber, roughly chopped
2 spring onions, roughly chopped
2 tsp chopped fresh basil, chives, marjoram or thyme
a pinch of salt
freshly ground black pepper
ice cubes, to serve (optional)

Plunge the tomatoes into boiling water for 30 seconds, then refresh in cold water. Peel away the skins. Halve the tomatoes and remove the seeds.

Put all the ingredients in a blender or food processor and blend until the soup is perfectly smooth. Serve well chilled with two or three ice cubes floating in each, if you like.

Fillet of Beef with Asparagus

SERVES 4

450g (1lb) fillet beef steak, cut into 4 steaks
½ tsp olive oil
½ tsp rapeseed oil
10 asparagus spears, lightly steamed, to serve
green salad, to serve

Preheat the grill to medium. Smear the steak with the oils and grill for 2 minutes on each side for rare steak, or longer if you prefer your steak medium or well done.

Serve with the asparagus and a green salad.

Turkey Curry

SERVES 4

rapeseed oil, for frying
4 portions of turkey breast, about 125g (4½oz) each
Curry Sauce (see page 221)
2 ready-to-eat dried apricots, chopped
a pinch of salt
freshly ground black pepper
lightly steamed green beans, to serve

Put a smear of oil in a non-stick frying pan over a medium heat and gently fry the turkey pieces for 10–15 minutes until cooked through and the juices run clear.

Add the curry sauce and simmer gently for 2 minutes. Taste the sauce and add salt and pepper as needed. Add the apricots and stir gently, adding a little water if needed to make a pouring sauce. Serve with green beans.

Curry Sauce

2 tsp olive oil or rapeseed oil

2 onions, chopped

2 garlic cloves, chopped

600ml (20fl oz/1 pint) chicken or vegetable stock or water

1cm (½in) fresh root ginger, finely grated

1 tsp ground cumin

1 tsp ground turmeric

1 tsp cardamom pods

1 cinnamon stick

2 cloves

2 tsp ground coriander

2 tsp chopped fresh coriander

1 tsp chopped fresh parsley

1 red chilli, deseeded and finely chopped

½ tsp ordinary curry powder

125g carton low-fat natural yoghurt (optional)

(Quantities of each of the above ingredients depend entirely on personal taste.)

Heat the oil in a pan over a medium heat and cook the onions and garlic for 5 minutes or until softened. Empty the onion mixture into a colander with a dish underneath. Cover with clingfilm and leave to stand overnight. Do not chill.

Next day, fill a small pan three-quarters full with stock or water and put in all the ingredients except the onion and garlic and the yoghurt. Bring to the boil over a high heat and boil until only half the liquid remains, then add the onion and garlic. Put everything into a blender and process to a purée. If the sauce is too thin, boil it to reduce it further. If it is too thick, add more stock or water. Adjust the flavour to your liking, adding spices as needed. Add the yoghurt, if using.

You now have a low-calorie curry sauce, and your diet will allow you to enjoy as much as you wish.

Grilled Salmon with Spinach

SERVES 4

2 tsp olive oil

4 tsp lemon juice

1 tsp chopped fresh dill or a pinch of dried dill

4 portions of salmon fillet or steaks about 175g (6oz) each

a pinch of salt

freshly ground black pepper

a bunch of spinach leaves according to taste

Put the oil, lemon juice, dill and seasoning in a small bowl and mix well, then spread this over the top of the salmon.

Preheat the grill to medium and put the fish in a grill pan or baking tray. Grill for 8–10 minutes until cooked through and the fish flakes using a knife. Do not over-cook.

Put the spinach in a pan and cook over a medium-low heat with only the water that clings to the leaves, stirring occasionally, until tender but still bright green. Drain and serve with the salmon.

Mexican Beef Stir-fry

SERVES 4

450g (1lb) rump steak, cut into thin slices

1 large or 2 small courgettes, cut into strips

10 strips of pimiento (cherry pepper) or 1 red pepper, deseeded and sliced

1 small onion, sliced

a pinch of dried chilli flakes, or to taste

1 tbsp fresh chopped parsley
a pinch of salt
freshly ground black pepper
mixed green salad, to serve

Using a non-stick frying pan over a medium heat, dry-fry the beef for 3 minutes, then add the courgettes, pimiento, onion and chilli flakes.

Season with salt and pepper and add 2 tsp water, then cook, stirring continuously, until the vegetables and meat are tender. Stir in the parsley and serve with salad.

Herbed Plaice with Broccoli

SERVES 4

4 plaice fillets
2 tsp olive oil
1 tsp English mustard
1 tbsp fresh chopped parsley
freshly ground black pepper
lightly steamed broccoli, to serve

Put the plaice in a baking tray. Put the oil, mustard and parsley in a bowl and mix to combine, then spread this evenly over the fish. Preheat the grill to medium and cook the fish for 5 minutes or until just cooked through. Serve with broccoli.

Tomato Soup

SERVES 6

680g (1½lb) tomatoes
1 tbsp olive oil
1 large onion, chopped
1 garlic clove, crushed
1.2 litres (2 pints) chicken stock
1 tsp granulated artificial sweetener (optional)
½ tsp dried basil
2 tbsp low-fat natural yoghurt
a pinch of salt
freshly ground black pepper

Plunge the tomatoes into boiling water for 30 seconds, then refresh in cold water. Peel away the skins. Cut out the cores and chop the flesh.

Heat the oil in a large pan over medium heat, and gently fry the onion and garlic for 5 minutes. Add the tomatoes and cook for 2 minutes. Stir in the stock, sweetener, if using, and basil. Season with salt and pepper. Bring to the boil, then reduce the heat and simmer for 30 minutes. Blend the soup. Reheat in the pan and stir in the yoghurt.

Peanut Chicken

SERVES 4

4 tsp peanut butter
1 tbsp chopped fresh parsley
dried chilli flakes, to taste (optional)
4 skinless chicken breasts, about 125g (4½oz) each
lightly steamed sliced spring greens
a little olive oil and lemon juice, to serve (optional)

Preheat the oven to 180°C (160°C fan oven)/Gas 4. Put the peanut butter, parsley and chilli flakes in a small bowl and combine into a paste, then spread this over the chicken breasts.

Put into an ovenproof dish and bake for 15–20 minutes. Serve the chicken with the steamed greens dressed with a little olive oil and lemon juice, if you like.

Spiced Turkey with Courgettes

SERVES 4

4 portions of turkey breast, about 125g (4½oz) each
2 tbsp low-fat natural yoghurt
a pinch of ground cumin
a pinch of ground ginger
a pinch of ground cardamom
a pinch of ground coriander
½ garlic clove, crushed
a pinch of salt
freshly ground black pepper
lightly steamed sliced courgettes, to serve

Preheat the oven to 180°C (160°C fan oven)/Gas 4. Put the turkey portions between two sheets of greaseproof paper and use a rolling pin or the base of a frying pan to flatten them slightly into thick escalopes.

Put the yoghurt in a bowl and add the spices, garlic and seasoning. Use to spread over the turkey pieces. Put on a baking tray and cook in the oven for 10–15 minutes until cooked through and the juices run clear. Serve with the courgettes.

Prawns with Rocket Dressing and Asparagus

SERVES 2

10 raw king prawns, peeled and deveined

1 bunch of rocket leaves

1 tsp olive, rapeseed or sesame oil

1 garlic clove, crushed

a pinch of salt

freshly ground black pepper

10 lightly steamed asparagus spears, to serve

Put the prawns in a steamer over a pan of boiling water and steam until pink and cooked through. Do not over-cook.

Meanwhile, put the rocket leaves in a blender and add the oil, garlic, and salt and pepper. Process into a purée, adding a little water if needed. Serve the prawns on a bed of asparagus with the rocket dressing drizzled over.

Orientation Phase Lentil Soup

SERVES 6

2 tbsp olive oil

1 onion, chopped

2 garlic cloves, crushed

225g (8oz) red lentils

225g (8oz) tinned tomatoes

1.2 litres (2 pints) vegetable stock

a pinch of salt

freshly ground black pepper

chopped fresh parsley, to serve

wholegrain or sourdough bread, to serve

Heat the oil in a pan over a medium heat and gently fry the onion and garlic for 5 minutes. Add the remaining ingredients. Bring to the boil, then reduce the heat and simmer gently for 20 minutes or until the lentils are soft. Season and serve the soup as it is or, if you prefer, blend it until smooth. Sprinkle with parsley and serve with bread.

TIP

The soup can also be made with green or brown lentils and will take 45 minutes–1 hour to cook until tender.

Lentils are an excellent source of protein. Although they are relatively deficient in sulphur-containing amino-acids, they are rich in another essential amino-acid, lysine, in which many cereals are deficient. For this reason a combination of lentils and cereal provides a complete protein that compares well with animal protein. It is therefore a good idea to have a slice of wholegrain or sourdough bread with this soup.

Curried Pork Medallions

SERVES 4

rapeseed oil, for frying

650g (1lb 7oz) pork fillet (tenderloin), cut into medallions 2cm (¾in) thick

1 shallot or ½ small onion, chopped

1 tsp curry powder

2 ready-to-eat dried apricots, chopped

lightly steamed French or runner beans, to serve

Put a smear of oil in a non-stick frying pan over a medium heat and add the pork and shallot. Cook the pork gently for 3 minutes on each side or until lightly browned.

Add the curry powder and cook for a further 2 minutes. Add 3 tbsp water and simmer gently for 5 minutes or until the pork is cooked through. Stir in the apricots and add more water if needed to give you a smooth sauce. Serve with beans.

Ricotta Cheese Dessert

SERVES 1

100g (3½oz) low-fat ricotta cheese
1 tsp granulated artificial sweetener
½ tsp vanilla extract
a few toasted almonds or mini chocolate chips, to serve

Put all the ingredients in a bowl and mix together. Chill in the fridge until ready to serve. Serve with a sprinkling of almonds or chocolate chips.

ALTERNATIVE DINNER RECIPES

Shepherd's Pie

SERVES 4

2 tsp olive oil or rapeseed oil
2 onions, chopped
450g (1lb) lean minced beef
2 bay leaves
1 tbsp chopped fresh parsley, plus extra to garnish
Worcestershire sauce, to taste

2 courgettes, cut into chunks
a pinch of salt
freshly ground black pepper

Preheat the oven to 180°C (160°C fan oven) Gas 4. Heat the oil in a non-stick pan over a medium heat and cook the onions for 8 minutes or until light brown. Add the beef and the herbs, and salt and pepper to taste. Cook for 10 minutes or until brown, with no liquid left in the pan. Transfer to an ovenproof dish and sprinkle over the Worcestershire sauce.

Steam the courgettes until moderately soft, then transfer to a bowl. Crush the courgettes using a fork, then season to taste and spread over the beef. Bake for 25 minutes, then serve garnished with chopped parsley.

TIP

This recipe can be served with an additional vegetable of your choice. Remember that you can add herbs, spices or pepper to add more flavour, if you like.

Fish Curry

SERVES 2

225g (8oz) cod fillet, skinned and cut into strips
Curry Sauce (page 221)
cauliflower purée, to serve (see Tip)

Preheat the oven to 180°C (160°C fan oven)/Gas 4. Spread out the strips of cod evenly in an ovenproof dish. Cover with curry sauce, then cook in the oven for 10–15 minutes until tender. Serve with cauliflower purée.

> **TIP**
>
> Put cauliflower florets in a pan with ¼ chopped onion, ½ tsp mixed herbs and some ground black pepper. Pour in stock to come about 1.5cm (⅝ in) up the sides of the pan. Cook until tender, then drain and purée using a blender.

Grilled Tomato and Feta Salad

SERVES 1

2 tomatoes
25g (1oz) feta cheese, crumbled
a little olive oil, for drizzling
1 tsp chopped fresh oregano, or a pinch of dried oregano
freshly ground black pepper

Plunge the tomatoes into boiling water for 30 seconds, then refresh in cold water. Peel away the skins. Quarter the tomatoes and slice them into thick chunks.

Put a small piece of foil on a baking tray. Arrange half the tomato in a small circle and put the other half on top. Put the feta on top of the tomato. Preheat the grill to high. Grill the tomato mixture until the feta is golden brown. Slide on to a serving plate and sprinkle with olive oil, oregano and pepper.

> **TIP**
>
> This tasty Mediterranean-inspired dish is vegetarian (provided you choose a vegetarian feta) and it can be used either as a starter or main course.

Chapter Twenty-one

INTRODUCTION TO THE CONTINUATION PHASE

THIS IS THE PART FOR EVERYONE. Whether you are someone who has just finished the Orientation phase or you don't need to lose weight but simply want to follow a healthy diet, this is for you. There are no strict rules about what you may or may not eat. The main point is to be sensible about portion sizes and simply eat until you are no longer hungry. In the dinner menus you will find that vegetables are not generally specified for the main course. You can choose your own, following the guidelines earlier in this book; for example, a small portion of green vegetables and a couple of new potatoes – or something along those lines. The important points are small portions and healthy low-GI vegetables. But for those who want to shed more weight there are a few little tweaks.

TWEAK 1: GRAPEFRUIT

We have already looked at this in detail (see pages 199–200), but here is a brief recap. Recent research has shown that eating half a grapefruit before each main meal reduces the rise in blood sugar and keeps insulin levels low. This means that we feel less hungry, because high levels of insulin cause hunger and also stimulate the liver to manufacture fat, which increases body weight and also causes coronary heart disease.

If you still have weight to lose – and even if you haven't – grapefruit is almost a magical food. The reason that it is also good for those who don't need to lose weight is that, by keeping insulin levels low, grapefruit lowers the risk of heart disease and type-2 diabetes.

Unless you really don't like it, try to eat half a grapefruit before each meal. (But remember to see the warning about grapefruit interactions with certain medications in Appendix 2.)

TWEAK 2: PORTION SIZES

As previously mentioned, be sensible about portion sizes and simply eat until you are no longer hungry – but be careful! The key words are *until you are no longer hungry*. There is a difference between hunger and craving. So much of the excess food that we eat happens not because we are still hungry but because we *crave* that food. The huge portion of roast beef, the extra roast potatoes, the desserts – eating these has little to do with hunger, so we need to become more aware of hunger and to be able to distinguish it from craving.

Another way of reducing the amount of food we eat is to not start out each meal feeling ravenous. Feeling ravenous means that our blood sugar is low. A light snack between meals or shortly before a meal works wonders for this. Good examples are a slice of low-fat cheese, a piece of fruit or carrot, or a few nuts. It takes much less food to prevent a low blood sugar than it does to correct it.

What is a suitable portion size?

When considering the diet aspects of weight loss and weight control, portion size is very important. In fact, a common reason for having difficulty in losing or maintaining weight is portion sizes that are too large. Throughout this book, where no specific portion size is given, assume that a small portion is what is intended. But what is a small portion? Below is some guidance on recommended portion sizes and amounts for an average adult aiming to maintain his or her weight. The portion sizes and numbers are based on published guidelines that estimate an average person's nutritional and energy requirements.

Protein foods (meat, fish, eggs, beans, pulses, nuts)

This group is important for growth and repair. Try to include one portion in at least two of your meals each day. Count as one portion:

▶ 100g (3½oz) raw/75g (2¾oz) cooked lean meat (the size of a deck of cards).

▶ 75g (2¾oz) oily fish or 150g (5½oz) white fish (the size of a cheque book).

▶ 2 medium eggs.

▶ 4 tbsp pulses (a heaped handful), such as chickpeas or lentils.

▶ 2 tbsp (30g/1oz) nuts (a small handful) makes an ideal snack, but spread this amount throughout the day.

Starchy foods

These form our main source of energy and should be present in every meal. Count as one portion:

▶ One-third of a soup bowl.

▶ 2–3 small boiled potatoes.

▶ 1½ cups of boiled pasta (2 handfuls).

▶ ⅓ cup of boiled rice (3 heaped tbsp).

▶ 115g (4oz) cooked noodles (⅔ cup/1 handful).

▶ Half a pitta bread.

Dairy

Dairy foods are another good source of protein and provide calcium, which is important for healthy bones and teeth. Skimmed, semi-skimmed and low-fat versions contain as much calcium as the full versions. Count as one portion:

▶ 200ml (7fl oz/⅓ pint) of skimmed or semi-skimmed milk (a small glass).

▶ 150ml (5fl oz/¼ pint) low-fat or fat-free yoghurt (a small pot).

▶ 2 tbsp (90g/3¼oz) cottage cheese.

▶ 30g (1oz) hard cheese (the size of a small matchbox) as an occasional treat.

Fruit and vegetables

The current recommendation is to eat at least five portions a day. Recently some experts have advocated nine portions, but most people would find this a difficult target to achieve. Count as one portion:

▶ 80g (3oz) of any fruit or vegetable. Examples include:
  - 1–2 slices of large fruit, such as pineapple or mango.
  - 1 medium fruit, such as apple, banana, orange or peach.
  - 2 small fruits, such as satsumas, plums or kiwi fruits.
  - 1–2 handfuls of berries or grapes.
  - 150ml (5fl oz/¼ pint) (a small glass) of fruit juice or smoothie (but note that this is likely to be high in sugar).
  - 3 heaped tbsp vegetables, such as mixed vegetables, peas or carrots.
  - 1 soup bowl of salad leaves.
  - 150ml (5fl oz/¼ pint) (a small glass) of vegetable smoothie (but note that there is a limit of one smoothie, fruit or veggie, to count towards your 'five a day' of fruit and vegetables).

An easy way to cut down portion sizes

Use smaller plates or bowls for your meals. A small plate full of food is much more inviting than a large plate that is half empty.

The Continuation phase is for life. Initially, follow the recipe suggestions in this book, then, as you become more experienced and familiar with the recipes and cooking methods, you can start to devise your own menus.

If, for any reason, you find that your weight has increased again – no one is perfect! – go back to the Orientation Phase for a couple of weeks, and then return to Continuation.

Chapter Twenty-two

THE CONTINUATION PHASE DAILY MENUS

DAY 1

BREAKFAST

A glass of water

Optional: half a grapefruit (with optional artificial sweetener)

Choose from the following foods:

an approved breakfast cereal (see pages 189–90)

low-fat plain yoghurt

low-fat fruit yoghurt

2 scrambled eggs on wholegrain toast

poached egg with grilled lean back bacon,
tomato and grilled mushrooms

2 boiled eggs with wholegrain toast 'soldiers'

Tea or decaffeinated coffee with optional skimmed milk
and sweetener, but no sugar

▶

MORNING SNACK

A glass of water

Choose from the following foods:

vegetable sticks (such as carrots, celery, cauliflower)

celery stick with low-fat cheese such as cottage,
Laughing Cow light cheese

celery stick or apple with 1 tsp peanut butter

low-fat sugar-free yoghurt

nuts (within the daily permitted quantity – see chart
'Orientation – foods to include and foods to avoid' on page 196)

Tea or decaffeinated coffee with optional skimmed milk
and sweetener, but no sugar

LUNCH

A glass of water

Optional: half a grapefruit (with optional artificial sweetener)

Stuffed Peppers*

AFTERNOON SNACK

A glass of water

Choose from the following foods:

vegetable sticks (such as carrots, celery, cauliflower)

celery stick with low-fat cheese, such as cottage,
Laughing Cow light cheese

celery stick or apple with 1 tsp peanut butter

low-fat sugar-free yoghurt

Nuts (within the daily permitted quantity – see chart
'Orientation – foods to include and foods to avoid' on page 196)

Tea or decaffeinated coffee with optional skimmed milk
and sweetener, but no sugar

DINNER

A glass of water

Optional: half a grapefruit (with optional artificial sweetener)

Lemon Chicken*

Fruit Pavlova (or Slimmers' Meringue)*

DAY 2

BREAKFAST

A glass of water

Optional: half a grapefruit (with optional artificial sweetener)

Choose from the following foods:

an approved breakfast cereal (see pages 189–90)

low-fat plain yoghurt

low-fat fruit yoghurt

scrambled egg on wholegrain toast

poached egg with grilled lean back bacon, tomato and grilled mushrooms

2 boiled eggs with wholegrain toast 'soldiers'

Tea or decaffeinated coffee with optional skimmed milk and sweetener, but no sugar

MORNING SNACK

A glass of water

Choose from the following foods:

vegetable sticks (such as carrots, celery, cauliflower)

celery stick with low-fat cheese such as cottage, Laughing Cow light cheese

celery stick or apple with 1 tsp peanut butter

low-fat sugar-free yoghurt

nuts (within the daily permitted quantity – see chart 'Orientation – foods to include and foods to avoid' on page 196)

Tea or decaffeinated coffee with optional skimmed milk and sweetener, but no sugar

▶

LUNCH

A glass of water

Optional: half a grapefruit (with optional artificial sweetener)

Ham and low-fat cheese sandwich (such as
Laughing Cow light cheese),
using wholegrain or sourdough bread

You may add salad ingredients, if you wish

AFTERNOON SNACK

A glass of water

Choose from the following foods:

vegetable sticks (such as carrots, celery, cauliflower)

celery stick with low-fat cheese such as cottage,
Laughing Cow light cheese

celery stick or apple with 1 tsp peanut butter

low-fat sugar-free yoghurt

nuts (within the daily permitted quantity – see chart
'Orientation – foods to include and foods to avoid' on page 196)

Tea or decaffeinated coffee with optional skimmed milk
and sweetener, but no sugar

DINNER

A glass of water

Optional: half a grapefruit (with optional artificial sweetener)

Ginger Haddock Parcels*

Peach Melba*

DAY 3

BREAKFAST

A glass of water

Optional: half a grapefruit (with optional artificial sweetener)

Choose from the following foods:

an approved breakfast cereal (see pages 189–90)

low-fat plain yoghurt

low-fat fruit yoghurt

scrambled egg on wholegrain toast

poached egg with grilled lean back bacon, tomato and grilled mushrooms

2 boiled eggs with wholegrain toast 'soldiers'

Tea or decaffeinated coffee with optional skimmed milk and sweetener, but no sugar

MORNING SNACK

A glass of water

Choose from the following foods:

vegetable sticks (such as carrots, celery, cauliflower)

celery stick with low-fat cheese such as cottage, Laughing Cow light cheese

celery stick or apple with 1 tsp peanut butter

low-fat sugar-free yoghurt

nuts (within the daily permitted quantity – see chart 'Orientation – foods to include and foods to avoid' on page 196)

Tea or decaffeinated coffee with optional skimmed milk and sweetener, but no sugar

▶

LUNCH

A glass of water

Optional: half a grapefruit (with optional artificial sweetener)

Chicken and Pasta Salad*

AFTERNOON SNACK:

A glass of water

Choose from the following foods:

vegetable sticks (such as carrots, celery, cauliflower)

celery stick with low-fat cheese such as cottage,
Laughing Cow light cheese

celery stick or apple with 1 tsp peanut butter

low-fat sugar-free yoghurt

nuts (within the daily permitted quantity – see chart
'Orientation – foods to include and foods to avoid' on page 196)

Tea or decaffeinated coffee with optional skimmed or milk
and sweetener, but no sugar

DINNER

A glass of water

Optional: half a grapefruit (with optional artificial sweetener)

Curried Lamb*

Apple Mousse*

DAY 4

BREAKFAST

A glass of water

Optional: half a grapefruit (with optional artificial sweetener)

Choose from the following foods:

an approved breakfast cereal (see pages 189–90)

low-fat plain yoghurt

low-fat fruit yoghurt

scrambled egg on wholegrain toast

poached egg with grilled lean back bacon, tomato and grilled mushrooms

2 boiled eggs with wholegrain toast 'soldiers'

Tea or decaffeinated coffee with optional skimmed milk and sweetener, but no sugar

MORNING SNACK

A glass of water

Choose from the following foods:

vegetable sticks (such as carrots, celery, cauliflower)

celery stick with low-fat cheese such as cottage, Laughing Cow light cheese

celery stick or apple with 1 tsp peanut butter

low-fat sugar-free yoghurt

nuts (within the daily permitted quantity – see chart 'Orientation – foods to include and foods to avoid' on page 196)

Tea or decaffeinated coffee with optional skimmed milk and sweetener, but no sugar

▶

LUNCH

A glass of water

Optional: half a grapefruit (with optional artificial sweetener)

Beef and Pepper Kebabs*

AFTERNOON SNACK

A glass of water

Choose from the following foods:

vegetable sticks (such as carrots, celery, cauliflower)

celery stick with low-fat cheese such as cottage,
Laughing Cow light cheese

celery stick or apple with 1 tsp peanut butter

low-fat sugar-free yoghurt

nuts (within the daily permitted quantity – see chart
'Orientation – foods to include and foods to avoid' on page 196)

Tea or decaffeinated coffee with optional skimmed milk
and sweetener, but no sugar

DINNER

A glass of water

Optional: half a grapefruit (with optional artificial sweetener)

Rosemary-baked Chicken*

Orange Sorbet*

DAY 5

BREAKFAST

A glass of water

Optional: half a grapefruit (with optional artificial sweetener)

Choose from the following foods:

an approved breakfast cereal (see pages 189–90)

low-fat plain yoghurt

low-fat fruit yoghurt

scrambled egg on wholegrain toast

poached egg with grilled lean back bacon, tomato and
grilled mushrooms

2 boiled eggs with wholegrain toast 'soldiers'

Tea or decaffeinated coffee with optional skimmed milk
and sweetener, but no sugar

MORNING SNACK

A glass of water

Choose from the following foods:

vegetable sticks (such as carrots, celery, cauliflower)

celery stick with low-fat cheese such as cottage,
Laughing Cow light cheese

celery stick or apple with 1 tsp peanut butter

low-fat sugar-free yoghurt

nuts (within the daily permitted quantity – see chart
'Orientation – foods to include and foods to avoid' on page 196)

Tea or decaffeinated coffee with optional skimmed milk
and sweetener, but no sugar

▶

LUNCH

A glass of water

Optional: half a grapefruit (with optional artificial sweetener)

Tuna and Pasta Salad*

AFTERNOON SNACK

A glass of water

Choose from the following foods:

vegetable sticks (such as carrots, celery, cauliflower)

celery stick with low-fat cheese such as cottage,
Laughing Cow light cheese

celery stick or apple with 1 tsp peanut butter

low-fat sugar-free yoghurt

nuts (within the daily permitted quantity – see chart
'Orientation – foods to include and foods to avoid' on page 196)

Tea or decaffeinated coffee with optional skimmed milk
and sweetener, but no sugar

DINNER

A glass of water

Optional: half a grapefruit (with optional artificial sweetener)

Veal in Breadcrumbs*

Apple and Lemon Compote*

DAY 6

BREAKFAST

A glass of water

Optional: half a grapefruit (with optional artificial sweetener)

Choose from the following foods:

an approved breakfast cereal (see pages 189–90)

low-fat plain yoghurt

low-fat fruit yoghurt

scrambled egg on wholegrain toast

poached egg with grilled lean back bacon, tomato and grilled mushrooms

2 boiled eggs with wholegrain toast 'soldiers'

Tea or decaffeinated coffee with optional skimmed milk and sweetener, but no sugar

MORNING SNACK

A glass of water

Choose from the following foods:

vegetable sticks (such as carrots, celery, cauliflower)

celery stick with low-fat cheese such as cottage, Laughing Cow light cheese

celery stick or apple with 1 tsp peanut butter

low-fat sugar-free yoghurt

nuts (within the daily permitted quantity – see chart 'Orientation – foods to include and foods to avoid' on page 196)

Tea or decaffeinated coffee with optional skimmed milk and sweetener, but no sugar

▶

LUNCH

A glass of water

Optional: half a grapefruit (with optional artificial sweetener)

Tuna Salad* with Marinated Mushrooms*

AFTERNOON SNACK

A glass of water

Choose from the following foods:

vegetable sticks (such as carrots, celery, cauliflower)

celery stick with low-fat cheese such as cottage,
Laughing Cow light cheese

celery stick or apple with 1 tsp peanut butter

low-fat sugar-free yoghurt

nuts (within the daily permitted quantity – see chart
'Orientation – foods to include and foods to avoid' on page 196)

Tea or decaffeinated coffee with optional skimmed milk
and sweetener, but no sugar

DINNER

A glass of water

Optional: half a grapefruit (with optional artificial sweetener)

Chicken and Pepper Rice*

Raspberry Sorbet*

DAY 7

BREAKFAST

A glass of water

Optional: half a grapefruit (with optional artificial sweetener)

Choose from the following foods:

an approved breakfast cereal (see pages 189–90)

low-fat plain yoghurt

low-fat fruit yoghurt

scrambled egg on wholegrain toast

poached egg with grilled lean back bacon, tomato and grilled mushrooms

2 boiled eggs with wholegrain toast 'soldiers'

Tea or decaffeinated coffee with optional skimmed milk and sweetener, but no sugar

MORNING SNACK

A glass of water

Choose from the following foods:

vegetable sticks (such as carrots, celery, cauliflower)

celery stick with low-fat cheese such as cottage, Laughing Cow light cheese

celery stick or apple with 1 tsp peanut butter

low-fat sugar-free yoghurt

nuts (within the daily permitted quantity – see chart 'Orientation – foods to include and foods to avoid' on page 196)

Tea or decaffeinated coffee with optional skimmed milk and sweetener, but no sugar

▶

LUNCH

A glass of water

Optional: half a grapefruit (with optional artificial sweetener)

Mushroom Torte*

AFTERNOON SNACK

A glass of water

Choose from the following foods:

vegetable sticks (such as carrots, celery, cauliflower)

celery stick with low-fat cheese such as cottage,
Laughing Cow light cheese

celery stick or apple with 1 tsp peanut butter

low-fat sugar-free yoghurt

nuts (within the daily permitted quantity – see chart
'Orientation – foods to include and foods to avoid' on page 196)

Tea or decaffeinated coffee with optional skimmed milk
and sweetener, but no sugar

DINNER

A glass of water

Optional: half a grapefruit (with optional artificial sweetener)

Roast Lamb with Garlic*

Chocolate Soufflé*

DAY 8

BREAKFAST

A glass of water

Optional: half a grapefruit (with optional artificial sweetener)

Choose from the following foods:

an approved breakfast cereal (see pages 189–90)

low-fat plain yoghurt

low-fat fruit yoghurt

2 scrambled eggs on wholegrain toast

poached egg with grilled lean back bacon, tomato and grilled mushrooms

2 boiled eggs with wholegrain toast 'soldiers'

Tea or decaffeinated coffee with optional skimmed milk and sweetener, but no sugar

MORNING SNACK

A glass of water

Choose from the following foods:

vegetable sticks (such as carrots, celery, cauliflower)

celery stick with low-fat cheese such as cottage, Laughing Cow light cheese

celery stick or apple with 1 tsp peanut butter

low-fat sugar-free yoghurt

nuts (within the daily permitted quantity – see chart 'Orientation – foods to include and foods to avoid' on page 196)

Tea or decaffeinated coffee with optional skimmed milk and sweetener, but no sugar

▶

LUNCH

A glass of water

Optional: half a grapefruit (with optional artificial sweetener)

Herbed Lamb Kebabs*

AFTERNOON SNACK

A glass of water

Choose from the following foods:

vegetable sticks (such as carrots, celery, cauliflower)

celery stick with low-fat cheese such as cottage,
Laughing Cow light cheese

celery stick or apple with 1 tsp peanut butter

low-fat sugar-free yoghurt

nuts (within the daily permitted quantity – see chart
'Orientation – foods to include and foods to avoid' on page 196)

Tea or decaffeinated coffee with optional skimmed milk
and sweetener, but no sugar

DINNER

A glass of water

Optional: half a grapefruit (with optional artificial sweetener)

Country Chicken Casserole* with basmati or wild rice

DAY 9

BREAKFAST

A glass of water

Optional: half a grapefruit (with optional artificial sweetener)

Choose from the following foods:

an approved breakfast cereal (see pages 189–90)

low-fat plain yoghurt

low-fat fruit yoghurt

2 scrambled eggs on wholegrain toast

poached egg with grilled lean back bacon, tomato and grilled mushrooms

2 boiled eggs with wholegrain toast 'soldiers'

Tea or decaffeinated coffee with optional skimmed milk and sweetener, but no sugar

MORNING SNACK

A glass of water

Choose from the following foods:

vegetable sticks (such as carrots, celery, cauliflower)

celery stick with low-fat cheese such as cottage, Laughing Cow light cheese

celery stick or apple with 1 tsp peanut butter

low-fat sugar-free yoghurt

nuts (within the daily permitted quantity – see chart 'Orientation – foods to include and foods to avoid' on page 196)

Tea or decaffeinated coffee with optional skimmed milk and sweetener, but no sugar

▶

LUNCH

A glass of water

Optional: half a grapefruit (with optional artificial sweetener)

Carrot Soup*

Crunchy Red Cabbage Salad*

AFTERNOON SNACK

A glass of water

Choose from the following foods:

vegetable sticks (such as carrots, celery, cauliflower)

celery stick with low-fat cheese such as cottage,
Laughing Cow light cheese

celery stick or apple with 1 tsp peanut butter

low-fat sugar-free yoghurt

nuts (within the daily permitted quantity – see chart
'Orientation – foods to include and foods to avoid' on page 196)

Tea or decaffeinated coffee with optional skimmed milk
and sweetener, but no sugar

DINNER

A glass of water

Optional: half a grapefruit (with optional artificial sweetener)

Cod with Cucumber*

Baked Citrus Rhubarb*

DAY 10

BREAKFAST

A glass of water

Optional: half a grapefruit (with optional artificial sweetener)

Choose from the following foods:

an approved breakfast cereal (see pages 189–90)

low-fat plain yoghurt

low-fat fruit yoghurt

2 scrambled eggs on wholegrain toast

poached egg with grilled lean back bacon, tomato and grilled mushrooms

2 boiled eggs with wholegrain toast 'soldiers'

Tea or decaffeinated coffee with optional skimmed milk and sweetener, but no sugar

MORNING SNACK

A glass of water

Choose from the following foods:

vegetable sticks (such as carrots, celery, cauliflower)

celery stick with low-fat cheese such as cottage, Laughing Cow light cheese

celery stick or apple with 1 tsp peanut butter

low-fat sugar-free yoghurt

nuts (within the daily permitted quantity – see chart 'Orientation – foods to include and foods to avoid' on page 196)

Tea or decaffeinated coffee with optional skimmed milk and sweetener, but no sugar

▶

LUNCH

A glass of water

Optional: half a grapefruit (with optional artificial sweetener)

Mixed Vegetable Curry*

AFTERNOON SNACK

A glass of water

Choose from the following foods:

vegetable sticks (such as carrots, celery, cauliflower)

celery stick with low-fat cheese such as cottage,
Laughing Cow light cheese

celery stick or apple with 1 tsp peanut butter

low-fat sugar-free yoghurt

nuts (within the daily permitted quantity – see chart
'Orientation – foods to include and foods to avoid' on page 196)

Tea or decaffeinated coffee with optional skimmed milk
and sweetener, but no sugar

DINNER

A glass of water

Optional: half a grapefruit (with optional artificial sweetener)

Peppery Chicken and Herb Pasta*

Plum and Pear Compote*

DAY 11

BREAKFAST

A glass of water

Optional: half a grapefruit (with optional artificial sweetener)

Choose from the following foods:

an approved breakfast cereal (see pages 189–90)

low-fat plain yoghurt

low-fat fruit yoghurt

2 scrambled eggs on wholegrain toast

poached egg with grilled lean back bacon, tomato and grilled mushrooms

2 boiled eggs with wholegrain toast 'soldiers'

Tea or decaffeinated coffee with optional skimmed milk and sweetener, but no sugar

MORNING SNACK

A glass of water

Choose from the following foods:

vegetable sticks (such as carrots, celery, cauliflower)

celery stick with low-fat cheese such as cottage, Laughing Cow light cheese

celery stick or apple with 1 tsp peanut butter

low-fat sugar-free yoghurt

nuts (within the daily permitted quantity – see chart 'Orientation – foods to include and foods to avoid' on page 196)

Tea or decaffeinated coffee with optional skimmed milk and sweetener, but no sugar

▶

LUNCH

A glass of water

Optional: half a grapefruit (with optional artificial sweetener)

Continuation Phase Lentil Soup*

Celery, Radish and Green Pepper Salad*

AFTERNOON SNACK

A glass of water

Choose from the following foods:

vegetable sticks (such as carrots, celery, cauliflower)

celery stick with low-fat cheese such as cottage,
Laughing Cow light cheese

celery stick or apple with 1 tsp peanut butter

low-fat sugar-free yoghurt

nuts (within the daily permitted quantity – see chart
'Orientation – foods to include and foods to avoid' on page 196)

Tea or decaffeinated coffee with optional skimmed milk
and sweetener, but no sugar

DINNER

A glass of water

Optional: half a grapefruit (with optional artificial sweetener)

Grilled Sole with Grapes*

Apple and Blackberry Compote*

DAY 12

BREAKFAST

A glass of water

Optional: half a grapefruit (with optional artificial sweetener)

Choose from the following foods:

an approved breakfast cereal (see pages 189–90)

low-fat plain yoghurt

low-fat fruit yoghurt

2 scrambled eggs on wholegrain toast

poached egg with grilled lean back bacon, tomato and grilled mushrooms

2 boiled eggs with wholegrain toast 'soldiers'

Tea or decaffeinated coffee with optional skimmed milk and sweetener, but no sugar

MORNING SNACK

A glass of water

Choose from the following foods:

vegetable sticks (such as carrots, celery, cauliflower)

celery stick with low-fat cheese such as cottage, Laughing Cow light cheese

celery stick or apple with 1 tsp peanut butter

low-fat sugar-free yoghurt

nuts (within the daily permitted quantity – see chart 'Orientation – foods to include and foods to avoid' on page 196)

Tea or decaffeinated coffee with optional skimmed milk and sweetener, but no sugar

▶

LUNCH

A glass of water

Optional: half a grapefruit (with optional artificial sweetener)

French Onion Soup*

Red Pepper and Beansprout Salad*

AFTERNOON SNACK

A glass of water

Choose from the following foods:

vegetable sticks (such as carrots, celery, cauliflower)

celery stick with low-fat cheese such as cottage,
Laughing Cow light cheese

celery stick or apple with 1 tsp peanut butter

low-fat sugar-free yoghurt

nuts (within the daily permitted quantity – see chart
'Orientation – foods to include and foods to avoid' on page 196)

Tea or decaffeinated coffee with optional skimmed milk
and sweetener, but no sugar

DINNER

A glass of water

Optional: half a grapefruit (with optional artificial sweetener)

Chicken Curry*

Lemon and Banana Jelly *

DAY 13

BREAKFAST

A glass of water

Optional: half a grapefruit (with optional artificial sweetener)

Choose from the following foods:

an approved breakfast cereal (see pages 189–90)

low-fat plain yoghurt

low-fat fruit yoghurt

2 scrambled eggs on wholegrain toast

poached egg with grilled lean back bacon, tomato and grilled mushrooms

2 boiled eggs with wholegrain toast 'soldiers'

Tea or decaffeinated coffee with optional skimmed milk and sweetener, but no sugar

MORNING SNACK

A glass of water

Choose from the following foods:

vegetable sticks (such as carrots, celery, cauliflower)

celery stick with low-fat cheese such as cottage, Laughing Cow light cheese

celery stick or apple with 1 tsp peanut butter

low-fat sugar-free yoghurt

nuts (within the daily permitted quantity – see chart 'Orientation – foods to include and foods to avoid' on page 196)

Tea or decaffeinated coffee with optional skimmed milk and sweetener, but no sugar

▶

LUNCH

A glass of water

Optional: half a grapefruit (with optional artificial sweetener)

Chilli Bean and Frankfurter Salad*

AFTERNOON SNACK

A glass of water

Choose from the following foods:

vegetable sticks (such as carrots, celery, cauliflower)

celery stick with low-fat cheese such as cottage,
Laughing Cow light cheese

celery stick or apple with 1 tsp peanut butter

low-fat sugar-free yoghurt

nuts (within the daily permitted quantity – see chart
'Orientation – foods to include and foods to avoid' on page 196)

Tea or decaffeinated coffee with optional skimmed milk
and sweetener, but no sugar

DINNER

A glass of water

Optional: half a grapefruit (with optional artificial sweetener)

Haddock in Parsley Sauce*

Hot Fruit Compote*

DAY 14

BREAKFAST

A glass of water

Optional: half a grapefruit (with optional artificial sweetener)

Choose from the following foods:

an approved breakfast cereal (see pages 189–90)

low-fat plain yoghurt

low-fat fruit yoghurt

2 scrambled eggs on wholegrain toast

poached egg with grilled lean back bacon, tomato and grilled mushrooms

2 boiled eggs with wholegrain toast 'soldiers'

Tea or decaffeinated coffee with optional skimmed milk and sweetener, but no sugar

MORNING SNACK

A glass of water

Choose from the following foods:

vegetable sticks (such as carrots, celery, cauliflower)

celery stick with low-fat cheese such as cottage, Laughing Cow light cheese

celery stick or apple with 1 tsp peanut butter

low-fat sugar-free yoghurt

nuts (within the daily permitted quantity – see chart 'Orientation – foods to include and foods to avoid' on page 196)

Tea or decaffeinated coffee with optional skimmed milk and sweetener, but no sugar

▶

LUNCH

A glass of water

Optional: half a grapefruit (with optional artificial sweetener)

Celery Soup*

Cucumber Jelly*

AFTERNOON SNACK

A glass of water

Choose from the following foods:

vegetable sticks (such as carrots, celery, cauliflower)

celery stick with low-fat cheese such as cottage, Laughing Cow light cheese

celery stick or apple with 1 tsp peanut butter

low-fat sugar-free yoghurt

nuts (within the daily permitted quantity – see chart 'Orientation – foods to include and foods to avoid' on page 196)

Tea or decaffeinated coffee with optional skimmed milk and sweetener, but no sugar

DINNER

A glass of water

Optional: half a grapefruit (with optional artificial sweetener)

Roast Beef with Yorkshire Pudding*

Crêpes Suzette*

(Yes, you read the above correctly!
This menu is a little reward for you. But you will see that the dishes are prepared in a low-GI way.)

Chapter Twenty-three

RECIPES FOR THE CONTINUATION PHASE

THE RECIPES ARE IN THE order of the daily menus.

Stuffed Peppers

SERVES 4

350g (12oz) lean minced beef

2 small onions, finely chopped

2 carrots, grated

115g (4oz) mushrooms, chopped

2 garlic cloves, crushed

400g (14oz) can tomatoes, drained and juice reserved

1 tsp dried mixed herbs

4 green peppers, halved and deseeded

300ml (10fl oz/½ pint) stock

a pinch of salt

freshly ground black pepper

Preheat the oven to 180°C (160°C fan oven)/Gas 4. Put the beef in a non-stick frying pan over a medium heat and fry it in its own fat.

Drain off the fat from the beef and add the onions, carrots, mushrooms and garlic. Cook over a low heat for 10 minutes or until the onions are soft, then add the tomatoes, herbs, and salt and pepper.

Stuff the pepper halves with the beef mixture, then put them in an ovenproof dish and pour over the juice from the tomatoes and the stock. Cover and cook for 45 minutes or until the peppers are tender.

Lemon Chicken

SERVES 4

2 tbsp olive, rapeseed oil or sesame oil, plus extra for greasing
4 chicken breasts, about 125g (4½oz) each, with skin
4 tbsp lemon juice
zest of 1 lemon
2 garlic cloves, crushed
a pinch of salt
freshly ground black pepper
chopped parsley, to garnish

Preheat the oven to 180°C (160°C fan oven)/Gas 4 and grease a shallow ovenproof dish. Put the chicken breasts in the dish. Put the lemon juice, zest, oil and garlic in a small bowl and mix together.

Lightly sprinkle the chicken pieces with a little salt and pepper, then pour the lemon mixture evenly over the chicken. Cover with foil and bake for 45 minutes, basting occasionally. Remove the foil and cook for a further 15 minutes to allow the chicken to brown slightly. Before serving, remove the chicken skin and sprinkle with chopped parsley to garnish.

Fruit Pavlova (or Slimmers' Meringue)

SERVES 4

3 large egg whites

1 tsp cream of tartar

3 tbsp skimmed milk powder

2 tbsp granulated sweetener

1 large punnet of strawberries, hulled, or 400g (14oz) tin fruit
   salad in unsweetened syrup, drained

6 mint sprigs

Preheat the oven to 140°C (120°C fan oven)/Gas 1. On a sheet of baking parchment, draw a circle round a 20cm (8in) plate. Put this on the baking sheet with the circle underneath. Put the egg whites in a clean, grease-free bowl and start to whisk them.

Add the cream of tartar and continue to whisk until they form stiff peaks. Sprinkle over the skimmed milk powder and sweetener, and continue whisking until peaks form again.

Spread (or pipe) the mixture smoothly over the circle on the prepared baking sheet. Cook in the oven for 1 hour. Cool, then loosen carefully with a palette knife and transfer to a serving dish. Pile the fruit on top of the meringue, then top with the sprigs of mint.

Ginger Haddock Parcels

SERVES 4

4 haddock fillets, 175g (6oz) each, skinned

1½ tbsp lemon juice

½ tsp ground ginger

2 tsp soy sauce

2 tbsp olive oil, rapeseed oil or sesame oil

225g (8oz) mushrooms, sliced
a pinch of salt
freshly ground black pepper
boiled basmati rice and a green salad, to serve

Preheat the oven to 180°C (160°C fan oven)/Gas 4. Take 4 pieces of foil large enough to wrap around each fillet of haddock and put a fillet on each.

Put the lemon juice, ginger, soy sauce and oil in a small bowl and mix together. Put a quarter of the mixture on top of each fillet and then put the mushrooms on top. Season with salt and pepper, then fold over the foil to make four parcels. Bake for 20 minutes, or until cooked through and the fish flakes easily with a knife. Serve with rice and a salad.

Peach Melba

SERVES 2

275ml (9½fl oz) low-fat natural yoghurt
½ tsp liquid sweetener, plus extra for the purée, to taste
1 egg white
½ tsp vanilla extract
55g (2oz) raspberries
1 peach, sliced

Put the yoghurt and ½ tsp sweetener in a freezerproof container and stir together, then put in the freezer for 15 minutes to chill. Put the egg white in a clean, grease-free bowl and whisk until it forms soft peaks.

Spoon the yoghurt mixture into the bowl with the egg white and add the vanilla extract, then carefully fold together using a spatula. Tip back into the freezerproof container and freeze until firm.

Put the raspberries in a blender and process to make a smooth purée, then pass them through a sieve to remove the pips. Add a little sweetener to taste. Scoop out the frozen yoghurt, and serve with the purée and slices of peach.

Chicken and Pasta Salad

SERVES 4

115g (4oz) wholewheat or durum wheat pasta rings or shells
225g (8oz) cooked chicken, skin removed, cut into bite-sized pieces
2 red apples, diced
2 celery sticks, chopped
2 tbsp Low-GI Mayonnaise (see page 297)
1 tbsp natural low-fat yoghurt
a pinch of salt
freshly ground black pepper
lettuce, to serve

Cook the pasta according to the instructions on the packet until *al dente* (tender but with a bite in the centre). Put into a serving bowl and leave to cool.

Add the chicken to the bowl, followed by the apples and celery, then season with salt and pepper. Mix well.

Put the mayonnaise in a small bowl and stir in the yoghurt, then add this to the chicken mixture and stir well to coat. Serve on a bed of lettuce.

Curried Lamb

SERVES 4

olive oil or rapeseed oil, for frying
450g (1lb) lean lamb, cut into cubes
2 tsp tomato purée
1 large tomato, diced
2 tbsp chopped fresh coriander
1–2 red chillies, to taste, deseeded and chopped
Curry Sauce (see page 221)
boiled basmati or wild rice, to serve

Put a smear of oil in a large non-stick frying pan over a medium heat. Add the lamb and cook for 10 minutes or until browned.

Stir in the tomato purée, tomato, coriander and chillies. Cover and cook the lamb for 5 minutes.

Add the curry sauce and return to the boil, cover and reduce the heat to low. Simmer for 1–1½ hours or until the meat is tender. (Alternatively, this can be cooked in a casserole in the oven at 150°C (130°C fan oven)/Gas 2 for 2 hours. Or put all the ingredients into a slow cooker set on low and cook for 6 hours.) Serve with rice.

Apple Mousse

SERVES 4

450g (1lb) cooking apples, peeled, cored and cut into chunks
2 tbsp redcurrant jelly
1 egg white
a little ground cinnamon, to sprinkle

Put the apples in a pan and add 100ml (3½fl oz) water. Cover and cook over a medium-low heat for 10 minutes or until the apples have turned into a thick purée, stirring occasionally. Take the lid off towards the end of cooking if the mixture looks too liquid.

Stir in the redcurrant jelly, then transfer the mixture to a large bowl and leave to cool.

Put the egg white in a clean, grease-free bowl and whisk until it forms stiff peaks. Fold this into the apple mixture, then spoon the mixture into four glass serving bowls. Serve chilled with a little cinnamon sprinkled on top.

Beef and Pepper Kebabs

SERVES 4

225ml (8fl oz) tomato juice (unsweetened)

2 garlic cloves, crushed

1 tsp dried mixed herbs

1 tbsp soy sauce

450g (1lb) rump steak, trimmed of fat, cut into large cubes

2 onions, quartered

1 green pepper, deseeded and cut into eighths

1 red pepper, deseeded and cut into eighths

115g (4oz) button mushrooms

a pinch of salt

freshly ground black pepper

boiled new or sweet potatoes, or basmati rice, to serve

Put the tomato juice in a shallow dish and add the garlic, herbs, soy sauce, and salt and pepper. Mix together well. Add the meat and mix well. Cover with clingfilm, and leave in the fridge for 2–5 hours to marinate, turning the meat from time to time. Meanwhile, if using wooden skewers, soak four for 30 minutes.

Drain the steak, then thread it on to four wooden or metal skewers, alternating it with a piece of onion, a piece of pepper and a mushroom. Preheat the grill. Put the kebabs on the grill pan and grill for 15–20 minutes, turning regularly, until the meat is cooked thoroughly. (Alternatively cook the kebabs on a barbecue.) Serve with potatoes.

Rosemary-baked Chicken

SERVES 4

1½ tbsp chopped fresh rosemary or 2 tsp dried rosemary
4 skinless chicken breasts, about 125g (4½oz) each
a pinch of salt
freshly ground black pepper
boiled basmati rice or sweet potato and lightly steamed green
    vegetables, to serve

Preheat the oven to 190°C (170°C fan oven)/Gas 5. Rub the rosemary, salt and pepper into the chicken breasts.

Wrap the chicken in a piece of foil and put it in a baking tray. Bake for 1 hour or until cooked through and the juices run clear. Serve with rice and vegetables.

Orange Sorbet

SERVES 4

175ml (6fl oz) unsweetened orange juice
2 tbsp lemon juice
1 tsp liquid sweetener
1 egg white
twists of orange zest or sprigs of mint, to decorate

Put the orange juice in a jug and add the lemon juice, sweetener and 275ml (9½fl oz) water. Stir well, then pour into a shallow freezerproof container and freeze for 2 hours or until just beginning to firm up.

Remove from the freezer and tip the mixture into a bowl, then mash it with a fork until the crystals are broken down.

Put the egg white in a clean, grease-free bowl and whisk until it forms stiff peaks. Fold this into the orange mixture using a spatula. Return the mixture to the container and freeze for 4 hours or until firm.

Before serving, transfer the mixture to the fridge for 20 minutes to allow it to soften slightly. Serve scoops in glass dishes and decorate with a twist of orange or a sprig of mint.

Tuna and Pasta Salad

SERVES 4

> 115g (4oz) wholewheat pasta rings or shells
> 2 tbsp Low-GI Vinaigrette (see page 297)
> 100g (3½oz) tuna in brine, drained and flaked
> lettuce and radishes, to serve

Cook the wholewheat pasta according to the instructions on the packet, until *al dente* (tender but with a bite in the centre). Drain in a colander and refresh under cold running water. Tip into a serving bowl and leave to cool completely.

Add the vinaigrette to the bowl of pasta and toss to combine. Add the tuna and gently combine. Leave to chill in the fridge. Serve on a bed of lettuce with a few radishes to garnish.

Veal in Breadcrumbs

SERVES 2

> 2 egg whites, lightly beaten
> 55g (2oz) wholegrain or sourdough breadcrumbs
> 2 veal escalopes
> 50ml (2fl oz) olive oil, rapeseed oil or sesame oil
> ½ lemon, cut in half, to garnish

Put the egg whites into a shallow dish and put the breadcrumbs onto a plate. Dip the veal into the egg whites, then into the bread-crumbs, and press the breadcrumbs firmly into the meat. Put the coated escalopes onto a plate and leave to set in the fridge for 1 hour.

Heat the oil in a non-stick frying pan over medium-high heat and fry the veal for 5 minutes on each side. Serve garnished with a lemon wedge.

Apple and Lemon Compote

SERVES 4

> 450g (1lb) cooking apples, peeled, cored and cut into chunks
> 2 tbsp lemon juice
> 2 cloves
> liquid sweetener, to taste

Put the apples in a pan with the lemon juice, cloves, sweetener and 300ml (10fl oz/½ pint) water. Cover and cook over a medium-low heat for 10 minutes or until the apples have turned into a thick purée, stirring occasionally. Take the lid off towards the end of cooking if the mixture looks too liquid. Remove the cloves and serve hot or cold.

Tuna Salad

SERVES 4

> 1 lettuce
> 2 tomatoes, sliced
> ½ cucumber, sliced
> 185g tin tuna in brine
> 4 spring onions, chopped

Arrange a couple of lettuce leaves on each plate. Put the tomatoes and cucumber on top of the lettuce. Flake the tuna and divide it between each plate. Top with the spring onions.

> **TIP**
> Tuna in brine has much less fat compared to tuna in oil.

Marinated Mushrooms

SERVES 4

> 225g (8oz) button mushrooms, sliced
> 1 garlic clove, crushed
> 1 tbsp tomato purée
> 85m1 (3fl oz) white wine vinegar
> 1 tsp Worcestershire sauce
> ½ tsp mustard powder
> ½ tsp liquid sweetener
> a pinch of salt
> freshly ground black pepper
> 1 tbsp chopped fresh parsley, to serve

Put the mushrooms in a shallow bowl. Put all the remaining ingredients in a small bowl and add 50ml (2fl oz) water. Mix together well, then pour over the mushrooms. Cover with clingfilm and leave in the fridge for 7 hours or overnight to marinate, stirring the mushrooms occasionally.

Drain off the liquid, put the mushrooms into a serving dish and sprinkle with parsley.

TIP

This salad can be served either as a starter or as a salad accompaniment.

Chicken and Pepper Rice

SERVES 4

175g (6oz) basmati rice
2 tsp olive oil, rapeseed oil or sesame oil
1 medium onion, chopped
1 garlic clove, crushed
1 green pepper, deseeded and sliced
4 celery sticks, sliced
450g (1lb) cooked chicken breasts, skin removed, diced
115g (4oz) mushrooms, sliced
a pinch of salt
freshly ground black pepper
salad, to serve

Cook the rice as directed on the packet. Meanwhile, heat the oil in a non-stick frying pan over a medium heat and fry the onion and garlic for 3 minutes. Add the green pepper and celery, and cook for a further 5 minutes.

Add the chicken, mushrooms, and salt and pepper, then cover and cook gently for 5 minutes. When the rice is cooked, drain it and add it to the pan with the chicken mixture. Stir gently together. Serve with a salad.

Raspberry Sorbet

SERVES 4

> 450g (1lb) raspberries
> granulated or liquid sweetener, to taste
> 2 egg whites

Put all but 8 of the raspberries in a blender and process to form a purée. Push the purée through a sieve to remove the seeds. Sweeten to taste.

Put the egg whites in a clean, grease-free bowl and whisk until they form stiff peaks. Fold them into the purée using a spatula. Transfer to a shallow freezerproof container and freeze for 2 hours or until just beginning to firm up. Remove from the freezer and tip the mixture into a bowl, then mash it with a fork until the crystals are broken down.

Return the mixture to the container and freeze for 4 hours or until firm. Serve scoops in dessert glasses decorated with the remaining raspberries.

Mushroom Torte

SERVES 2

> 2 tsp olive oil, rapeseed oil or sesame oil, plus extra for greasing
> 1 medium onion, chopped
> 225g (8oz) mushrooms, chopped
> 2 large eggs
> 275ml (9½fl oz) skimmed milk
> a pinch of salt
> freshly ground black pepper

Preheat the oven to 180°C (160°C fan oven)/Gas 4 and lightly grease an ovenproof dish. Heat the oil in a non-stick pan over a medium heat, add the onion and cook for 5 minutes. Add the mushrooms and cook for 20 minutes, stirring occasionally.

Spread the mushrooms evenly over the base of the prepared dish. Put the eggs and milk in a bowl and whisk together, then season with salt and pepper. Pour the eggs over the mushrooms and bake for 35 minutes or until the centre is set.

TIPS

▶ This dish is similar to a quiche, but without the pastry.

▶ If you like, you can add a few sliced courgettes or chopped tomatoes – or any vegetable you prefer – before you add the eggs.

Roast Lamb with Garlic

SERVES 4

1.3kg (3lb) leg of lamb
2 garlic cloves, cut into slivers
1 tbsp fresh chopped rosemary or 1 tsp dried rosemary
1 tbsp fresh thyme or 1 tsp dried thyme
3 onions, sliced
2 sweet potatoes (cut into chunks) or 8–12 new potatoes, sliced
300ml (10fl oz/½ pint) hot meat stock
a pinch of salt
freshly ground black pepper
mint sauce, made with finely chopped fresh mint and vinegar

Preheat the oven to 230°C (210°C fan oven)/Gas 8. Using a sharp knife, make slits at 5cm (2in) intervals all over the lamb and insert the garlic into the slits. Rub the herbs all over the leg and put it in a roasting tin. Roast for 30 minutes.

Put the onions and potatoes in a large bowl and season with salt and pepper. Layer the potatoes and onions around the lamb. Pour the hot stock over the vegetables, and return the tin to the oven for a further 1½ hours, reducing the temperature to 200°C (180°C fan oven)/Gas 6 if the potatoes seem to be browning too quickly. Serve the lamb and vegetables with fresh mint sauce.

TIP

The vegetables will be full of flavour from the stock, making this a delicious way of serving a joint without having gravy.

Chocolate Soufflé

SERVES 4

425ml (15fl oz/¾ pint), plus 4 tbsp skimmed milk
2 tbsp cornflour
2 tbsp unsweetened cocoa powder
2 tsp liquid sweetener
1 tsp vanilla extract
3 egg whites
a little grated chocolate, to decorate

Heat the 425ml (15fl oz/¾ pint) skimmed milk in a pan over a medium heat. Put the cornflour in a small heatproof bowl and stir in the cocoa powder and sweetener with the 4 tbsp skimmed milk to form a smooth paste.

Gently stir a small amount of the warmed milk into the bowl, and then stir the mixture back into the pan. Cook, stirring continuously, until the mixture is thickened, then continue to cook for 3 minutes more to cook the cornflour. Add the vanilla, then pour the mixture into a large bowl and leave to cool.

Put the egg whites in a clean, grease-free bowl and whisk until they form stiff peaks. Fold into the cold chocolate mixture. Spoon the mixture into a serving dish and chill in the fridge. Serve decorated with grated chocolate.

Herbed Lamb Kebabs

SERVES 4

450g (1lb) leg of lamb, trimmed of fat and cut into large cubes
2 garlic cloves, crushed
1 tbsp chopped fresh mixed herbs or 1 tsp dried mixed herbs
juice of 2 lemons
1 onion, quartered
1 green pepper, deseeded and cut into eighths
4 small tomatoes
a pinch of salt
freshly ground black pepper
boiled new or sweet potatoes, or basmati rice, to serve

Put the lamb in a shallow dish, add the garlic and herbs, and season with salt and pepper. Pour the lemon juice over the mixture. Add the onion and pepper to the meat mixture and stir well. Cover with clingfilm and leave in the fridge for a 2–5 hours to marinate, turning the meat from time to time. Meanwhile, if using wooden skewers, soak four for 30 minutes.

Drain the lamb, then thread it on to four wooden or metal skewers, alternating it with a piece of onion and a piece of pepper. Put a tomato on to the end of each skewer. Preheat the grill. Put the kebabs on the grill pan and grill for 15–20 minutes, turning regularly, until the meat is cooked thoroughly. (Alternatively cook the kebabs on a barbecue.) Serve with potatoes.

Country Chicken Casserole

SERVES 4

1 tbsp olive oil or rapeseed oil

4 skinless chicken breasts, about 125g (4½oz) each

1 onion, sliced

450g (1lb) carrots, sliced

450g (1lb) leeks, sliced

4–6 small new potatoes, sliced

2 celery sticks, sliced

2 garlic cloves, crushed

600ml (20fl oz/1 pint) chicken stock

freshly ground black pepper

chopped fresh parsley, to garnish (optional)

Preheat the oven to 150°C (130°C fan oven)/Gas 2. Heat the oil in a large flameproof casserole over a medium-high heat. Fry the chicken breasts until golden. Remove from the pan and put on a plate.

Reduce the heat to medium and gently fry all the vegetables for 5 minutes. Stir in the garlic. Put the chicken back in the casserole on top of the vegetables. Pour the stock over the chicken and season with pepper. Cook in the oven for 2½ hours or until the chicken is cooked through and the juices run clear. Garnish with parsley, if using, before serving.

TIP

This dish needs no accompanying vegetables.

Carrot Soup

SERVES 4

> 1 tbsp olive oil
> 2 onions, chopped
> 450g (1lb) carrots, thinly sliced
> 1 garlic clove, crushed
> 850ml (1½ pints) beef stock
> 2 tbsp low-fat natural yoghurt
> a pinch of salt
> freshly ground black pepper

Heat the oil in a large pan over a medium heat. Add the vegetables and garlic, and cook for 5 minutes. Add the stock, salt and pepper. Bring to the boil and simmer for 20 minutes. Blend the soup, then reheat. Stir in the yoghurt before serving.

Crunchy Red Cabbage Salad

SERVES 4

> juice of ½ lemon
> 1 apple, cored and sliced
> 85g (3oz) red cabbage, shredded
> 3 celery sticks, chopped
> ½ green pepper, deseeded and chopped
> 2 tbsp low-fat natural yoghurt
> 1 tbsp Low-GI Mayonnaise (see page 297)

Put the lemon juice in a bowl and add the apple slices. Toss well to prevent discoloration. Lift out the apple and put it into a serving bowl.

Add the vegetables to the bowl followed by the yoghurt and mayonnaise, and toss well to mix thoroughly.

Cod with Cucumber

SERVES 4

> 4 cod steaks, about 175g (6oz) each
> zest and juice of 1 lemon
> 175g (6oz) cucumber, diced
> 55g (2oz) cottage cheese
> 140g (5oz) low-fat natural yoghurt
> a pinch of salt
> freshly ground black pepper
> sliced cucumber and chopped parsley, to garnish

Preheat the oven to 180°C (160°C fan oven)/Gas 4. Put the fish in a shallow ovenproof dish and sprinkle over the lemon zest and juice. Cover with foil and cook in the oven for 25 minutes. Drain off any excess liquid.

Put the cucumber in a small pan over a medium heat and add the cheese, yoghurt, and salt and pepper. Mix well and heat the mixture until warm, stirring. Serve on top of the fish, garnished with sliced cucumber and parsley.

Baked Citrus Rhubarb

SERVES 4

> 2 oranges
> 450g (1lb) rhubarb, cut into 2.5cm (1in) pieces
> liquid or granulated sweetener, if needed, to taste

Preheat the oven to 160°C (140°C fan oven)/Gas 3. Using a sharp knife, cut a thin slice of peel and pith from each end of an orange. Put cut side down on a plate and cut off the peel and pith in strips. Remove any remaining pith. Cut the orange into slices. Tip any juice on the plate into a small bowl. Repeat with the other orange.

Layer the rhubarb and oranges slices in an ovenproof dish. Drizzle over the reserved orange juice and cover with foil. Bake for 30 minutes or until the rhubarb is tender. Add the sweetener, if needed, when cooked. Serve hot or cold.

Mixed Vegetable Curry

SERVES 4

> 450g (1lb) mixed vegetables of your choice, such as diced
> aubergine, peppers, onions, carrots, celeriac, leeks, or
> cauliflower or broccoli cut into florets
> Curry Sauce (see page 221)
> boiled basmati or wild rice, to serve

If you are using cauliflower or broccoli florets, put these to one side. Put the remaining vegetables in a flameproof casserole or large, heavy-based pan and pour over the curry sauce. Bring to the boil over a medium heat, then reduce the heat and simmer for 20 minutes or until the vegetables are almost tender (the length of time will depend on the vegetables used).

Add the cauliflower or broccoli, if using, and cook for 10 minutes. Serve with rice.

RECIPES FOR THE CONTINUATION PHASE • 285

Peppery Chicken and Herb Pasta

SERVES 2

55g (2oz) pasta of your choice
2 tsp olive oil
100g (3½oz) skinless chicken breast, sliced
1 tbsp chopped fresh parsley
1 tbsp chopped fresh oregano
1 tsp Parmesan cheese
1 ready-to-eat dried apricot, chopped
freshly ground black pepper
green salad, to serve

Cook the pasta according to the packet instructions, al dente (tender but with a bite in the centre). Drain.

Meanwhile, heat the oil in a non-stick frying pan over a medium heat. Season the chicken with salt and plenty of pepper and add to the pan. Cook, stirring frequently, until cooked through and the juices run clear. Tip the pasta into the pan with the chicken and add the herbs, Parmesan and apricot. Adjust the seasoning if needed, and serve with salad.

Plum and Pear Compote

SERVES 4

225g (8oz) plums, halved and stoned
225g (8oz) pears, peeled, cored and sliced
liquid sweetener, to taste
a little cinnamon, to sprinkle

Put the plums in a pan and add the pears and 150ml (5fl oz/¼ pint) water. Cook over a medium heat until the fruit is tender. Add sweetener. Serve hot or cold with a sprinkling of cinnamon.

Continuation Phase Lentil Soup

SERVES 6

2 tsp olive oil or rapeseed oil
1 onion, chopped
2 garlic cloves, crushed
225g (8oz) red lentils
2 carrots, chopped
225g (8oz) tinned tomatoes
1.2 litres (2 pints) vegetable or chicken stock
a pinch of salt
freshly ground black pepper
chopped fresh parsley, to serve
wholegrain or sourdough bread, to serve

Heat the oil in a pan over a medium heat and gently fry the onion and garlic for 5 minutes. Add the remaining ingredients. Bring to the boil, then reduce the heat and simmer gently for 20 minutes. Season and serve the soup as it is or, if you prefer, blend it until smooth. Sprinkle with parsley and serve with bread.

TIP

The soup can also be made with green or brown lentils and will take 45 minutes–1 hour to cook. (see also Tip on lentils on page 227.)

Celery, Radish and Green Pepper Salad

SERVES 4

4 celery sticks, thinly sliced
12 radishes, thinly sliced
1 green pepper, deseeded and thinly sliced
1 tbsp Low-GI Vinaigrette (see page 297) or lemon juice

Mix the celery, radishes and green pepper in a serving bowl and add the vinaigrette or lemon juice. Toss to combine. Serve as a snack or as an accompaniment to snacks or main meals.

Grilled Sole with Grapes

SERVES 4

2 tbsp olive oil, rapeseed oil or sesame oil
4 lemon soles, about 175g (6oz) each
4 tbsp lemon juice
2 tbsp chopped fresh parsley
115g (4oz) green seedless grapes, halved
freshly ground black pepper
mixed salad and boiled new potatoes, to serve

Brush the oil over each sole and season with pepper. Preheat the grill. Put the sole on the grill pan or in a baking tray and grill for 10 minutes, turning once.

Meanwhile, put the lemon juice and chopped parsley in a small bowl and stir together. Serve the fish with the parsley mixture and grapes sprinkled over. Serve with salad and potatoes.

Apple and Blackberry Compote

SERVES 4

225g (8oz) apples, peeled, cored and sliced
225g (8oz) blackberries
liquid sweetener, to taste

Put the apples and blackberries in a pan and add 150ml (5fl oz/¼ pint) water. Cook over a medium heat until the fruit is tender. Add the sweetener. Serve hot or cold.

French Onion Soup

SERVES 4

1 tbsp olive oil, rapeseed oil or sesame oil
450g (1lb) onions, sliced
2 garlic cloves, crushed
½ tsp low-calorie granulated sweetener, to taste (optional)
850ml (l½ pints) beef stock
freshly ground black pepper
1 tbsp chopped fresh parsley

Heat the oil in a large pan over a medium heat and add the onions, garlic and sweetener, if using, then cover and cook over a low heat for 15 minutes until tender. Remove the lid and continue to cook until the onions start to brown.

Add the stock and bring to the boil, then cover and simmer gently for 30 minutes. Season to taste and sprinkle with parsley before serving.

Red Pepper and Beansprout Salad

SERVES 4

1 red pepper, deseeded and finely sliced
225g (8oz) beansprouts
2 tbsp Low-GI Vinaigrette (see page 297)

Put the pepper in a serving bowl and add the beansprouts. Add the vinaigrette and toss well to combine. Serve with a meat or fish dish.

Chicken Curry

SERVES 4

4 skinless chicken breasts, about 125g (4½oz) each, cut into
    bite-sized pieces
Curry Sauce (see page 221)
boiled basmati or wild rice, to serve

Put the chicken in a heavy-based pan over a medium heat and add the curry sauce. Bring to the boil, then reduce the heat and simmer gently for 15 minutes or until cooked through and the juices run clear. Serve with rice.

Lemon and Banana Jelly

SERVES 4

1 packet of sugar-free lemon jelly
juice of 1 lemon
1 banana

Make half the jelly according to the packet instructions. Stir in half the lemon juice and leave to cool. Pour into a jelly mould and leave to set in the fridge.

Make up the remaining jelly as before. Thinly slice the banana and arrange over the top of the jelly, then carefully pour the remaining jelly over the banana. Leave to set completely in the fridge. Unmould to serve.

Chilli Bean and Frankfurter Salad

SERVES 4

> 2 tomatoes
> 400g (14oz) tin red kidney beans, rinsed and drained
> 1 red pepper, deseeded and sliced
> 1 green pepper, deseeded and sliced
> 1 onion, thinly sliced
> 4 cooked Frankfurters, cut into bite-sized pieces
> chicory or lettuce, to serve
>
> **For the dressing:**
> 2 tbsp Low-GI Vinaigrette (see page 297)
> ½ tsp Tabasco sauce
> a pinch of chilli powder
> salt
> freshly ground black pepper

Plunge the tomatoes into boiling water for 30 seconds, then refresh in cold water. Peel away the skins. Core and chop the tomatoes roughly. Put all the ingredients into a large serving bowl.

Mix together the dressing ingredients and pour over the bean mixture. Stir well and chill in the fridge. Serve on a bed of lettuce or chicory.

Haddock in Parsley Sauce

SERVES 4

4 haddock fillets, about 175g (6oz) each
280g (10oz) low-fat natural yoghurt
4 tsp lemon juice
4 tbsp chopped fresh parsley
a pinch of salt
freshly ground black pepper

Pour boiling water into a frying pan to a depth of 3cm (1¼in) and bring to the boil over a high heat. Reduce the heat and add the fish. Simmer for 10 minutes or until tender.

Meanwhile, to make the sauce put the yoghurt and lemon juice in a small pan over a medium heat and carefully heat, but do not allow to boil. Season the mixture and add the chopped parsley. Gently lift out the fish using a slotted fish slice and serve with the sauce spooned over.

> **TIP**
> The fish can also be grilled for 10–15 minutes, if you prefer.

Hot Fruit Compote

SERVES 4

2 large oranges
2 large pears, peeled, cored and sliced
1 apple, peeled, cored and sliced
225g (8oz) fresh or frozen raspberries
liquid sweetener, to taste

a dash of cinnamon
low-fat natural yoghurt or custard made with skimmed milk
and artificial sweetener, to serve

Using a sharp knife, cut a thin slice of peel and pith from each end of an orange. Put cut side down on a plate and cut off the peel and pith in strips. Remove any remaining pith. Cut out each segment leaving the membrane behind. Squeeze the remaining juice from the membrane into a bowl. Repeat with the other orange.

Put the fruit and reserved orange juice in a pan with 150ml (5fl oz/¼ pint) water and cook gently for 10 minutes, then add the sweetener and a little cinnamon. Serve hot with yoghurt.

Celery Soup

Serves 2
1 tbsp olive oil
1 head of celery, chopped
600ml (20fl oz/1 pint) beef, chicken or vegetable stock
2 tbsp low-fat natural yoghurt
1 tbsp chopped fresh parsley
freshly ground black pepper

Put the oil in a large pan over a medium heat and cook the celery for 5 minutes. Add the stock and cook for 30 minutes or until tender.

Use a blender to process until smooth then stir in the yoghurt and parsley. Season with pepper.

TIP

If you're making stock with stock cubes, you will need 2 beef, chicken or vegetable stock cubes for this recipe.

Cucumber Jelly

SERVES 6

1 cucumber
15g sachet powdered gelatine
zest and juice of 2 lemons
280g (10oz) low-fat natural yoghurt
1 tsp chopped fresh mint
1 tsp chopped fresh thyme
a pinch of salt
freshly ground black pepper
lettuce, to serve (optional)

Cut 2.5cm (1in) off the end of the cucumber, then thinly slice it and arrange the slices in the base of a glass bowl. Peel the remaining cucumber and cut it into dice. Set aside.

Put the gelatine in a small heatproof bowl and add 150ml (5floz/¼ pint) cold water, then leave to soak up the liquid. Rest the bowl over a pan of simmering water and leave it to dissolve, stirring occasionally. Remove from the heat and stir in the lemon zest and juice.

Pour a thin layer of this lemon jelly into the glass bowl with the cucumber slices, then leave to set. Return the remainder of the lemon jelly to the hot water, and stir it from time to time so that it does not set.

When the bottom layer of the jelly is set, whisk the yoghurt into the gelatine mixture, then stir in the cucumber, mint and thyme. Season with salt and pepper. Pour the mixture into the glass bowl and leave to set. To serve, dip the bowl in hot water and turn the jelly on to a plate. Serve with lettuce, if you like.

Roast Beef and Yorkshire Pudding

SERVES 6

1 carrot, roughly chopped

1 celery stick, roughly chopped

3 fresh thyme sprigs, broken

1 rosemary sprig, roughly chopped

1 onion, roughly chopped

3 garlic cloves, peeled and left whole

1.5kg (3lb 5oz) beef topside

a pinch of salt

freshly ground black pepper

horseradish sauce, to serve

For the Yorkshire pudding

115g (4oz) wholemeal flour

300ml (10fl oz/½ pint) skimmed milk

1 egg

1 tbsp olive oil or rapeseed oil

a pinch of salt

Preheat the oven to 220°C (200°C fan oven)/Gas 7. Put all the vegetables, herbs and the garlic in a roasting tin and lay the beef on top. Season with salt and pepper. Roast for 1–1¼ hours according to your preference for rare or well-done meat. Leave the meat to rest for 10 minutes before carving. (The vegetables will caramelise and are for flavouring only.)

Meanwhile, to make the Yorkshire puddings, sift the flour and salt into a large jug, add the milk and egg, and stir to make a smooth batter. (Alternatively, put the ingredients in a blender or food processer and pulse a few times to combine.)

When the beef has been cooking for 50 minutes, put the oil in a Yorkshire pudding tin or a 12-cup cake tin and heat in the oven until the fat is hot. Add the batter to the pudding tin, or divide the batter among the cups, and cook in the oven for 30 minutes for a single pudding or 20 minutes for individual puddings, or until risen and golden brown. Serve the beef with the Yorkshire pudding and horseradish sauce.

TIP

Roasted meats, without any added fats, so beloved in many cookery books, are easy to cook and are an excellent way of preparing meat because some of the fat is lost during the cooking. Roast beef, served with horseradish sauce and low-GI wholemeal Yorkshire pudding is delicious.

Crêpes Suzette

SERVES 4 TO 6, DEPENDING ON GREED

55g (2oz) plain flour
55g (2oz) plain wholemeal flour
6 tbsp granulated artificial sweetener
300ml (10fl oz/½ pint) skimmed milk
1 egg
2 tbsp olive oil
85g (3oz) polyunsaturated margarine
finely grated zest of 2 oranges
2 tbsp Cointreau or Grand Marnier
1 tbsp brandy

Sift the flours into a large jug and add 3 tbsp of the sweetener. Add the milk and egg, and whisk just enough to make a smooth batter. (Alternatively, put the ingredients in a blender or food processer and pulse a few times to combine.)

Heat an 18cm (7in) non-stick frying pan over a high heat. Very lightly oil the pan and pour in a thin layer of batter to just coat the base of the pan, tilting the pan to spread it. Cook for 1 minute or until golden underneath.

Turn the pancake over using a palette knife. Cook the other side for 1 minute or until golden. Repeat with the remaining batter. Stack the crêpes between pieces of greaseproof paper to prevent them sticking together and keep warm while you cook the remainder. You should get 12 pancakes. Meanwhile, preheat the oven to 220°C (200°C fan oven) Gas 7.

To make the Suzette sauce, put the margarine in a bowl and add the remaining sweetener, the orange zest and Cointreau. Spread the mixture evenly over each pancake and fold each up into quarters. Put the pancakes in an ovenproof dish and put in the oven for 10 minutes to heat through.

Heat a ladle when ready to serve. Take the dish of crêpes to the table, pour on the brandy, and carefully ignite (this is best done with the room lights switched off). Spoon the liqueur and sauce over the pancakes, and serve.

TIP

Why this is a good version of the dish?

▶ It uses skimmed milk instead of whole milk.

▶ Artificial sweetener replaces sugar.

▶ It uses part wholemeal flour instead of all plain flour.

It is important to indulge in 'forbidden' foods occasionally, but at the same time it makes sense to do so in the healthiest way possible. This dish is one of my own favourites and is always a great hit at dinner parties.

Low-GI Mayonnaise

300ml (10fl oz/½ pint) skimmed milk
15g (½oz) cornflour
1½ tsp dry mustard
1 tsp paprika
12 drops of liquid sweetener
a pinch of salt
6 tbsp extra virgin olive oil
6 tbsp vinegar or lemon juice

Put the milk in a pan and add the cornflour, then stir together to make a paste. Cook over a medium heat until thickened.

Transfer the paste to a bowl and add the mustard, paprika, sweetener and salt, then beat the ingredients together until smooth. Gradually add the oil and vinegar, beating constantly, until the mixture is blended.

Low-GL Vinaigrette

3 tbsp wine vinegar
1 tbsp extra virgin olive oil
1 tsp Worcestershire sauce
2 tsp dry mustard
2 drops liquid sweetener

Put all the ingredients in a screw-top jar and shake well to combine.

Chapter Twenty-four

SOME COMMON CARBOHYDRATE FOODS AND THEIR GI VALUES

YOU WILL FIND YOURSELF referring to this chapter time and again, so it's important to bear several points in mind.

► First, in the LOW GI column, foods in CAPITALS have especially low GI values.

► Second, some foods, although with low GI values, have amounts of fat that exceed the recommended guidelines.

► Third, *only carbohydrates have GI values*, so meat, for example, which is made of protein and fat but contains no carbohydrate, has no GI value.

► Fourth – and this is the most important – the GI value of a food is not the be-all-and-end-all. Watermelon, for example, has a high GI, but combine it with several other fruits with low GI values and the overall GI value of such a fruit salad is low. The overall value of a combination of foods is called its glycemic load or GL (as we saw in Chapter 8).Christmas Party B.pdf

Another way to reduce the overall glycemic load of a meal is to combine carbohydrates with non-carbohydrates; for example, spaghetti on its own or with a tomato-based sauce has a higher glycemic load than spaghetti Bolognese. This is because the meat has no GI. In fact, it is very important to try to combine protein with carbohydrate as much as you can. Protein is slowly digested, which both reduces the glycemic load of the meal and also satisfies hunger more easily. This is one reason why high-protein diets help weight loss – you actually feel less hungry.

Finally, remember that the GI values in the next few pages are approximate. The GI value of a fruit, for example, will vary with its ripeness. The GI value of pasta will depend on how well cooked it is. So GI is not an exact science, but it is a good guide. If you use it sensibly it will help you both to control your weight and to eat a diet that is kind to your heart and your body's metabolism.

GI VALUES OF SOME COMMON CARBOHYDRATE FOODS

	Low GI	Medium GI	High GI
Biscuits	Oats	Shortbread	Morning coffee
Breads	Pumpernickel Sourdough 100% stoneground wholemeal	Croissant (contains significant fat) Crumpet Pitta bread, wholemeal Rye Wholemeal, not stoneground	Bagel Baguette Dark rye Gluten-free Melba toast White Wholemeal bread
Cereals	ALL-BRAN Muesli, toasted Porridge (not instant) Special K	Mini Wheats Muesli, natural Nutri-grain Porridge (instant)	Bran Flakes Coco Pops Cornflakes Grapenuts Rice Krispies Shredded Wheat Sultana Bran Weetabix

▶

	Low GI	Medium GI	High GI
Confectionery	Chocolate (contains significant fat)	Mars bar (contains significant fat) Muesli bar (contains significant fat)	Jelly beans
Convenience foods	Fish fingers SAUSAGES (contain significant fat)		
Crackers		Ryvita	Crispbread Rice cakes Water crackers
Dairy	Custard Ice cream, low-fat Milk, whole, semi-skimmed or skimmed Soya milk Yoghurt, with sugar, with or without fruit Yoghurt, with sweetener, with or without fruit	Condensed milk, sweetened Ice cream, full-fat	
Fruit	Apple Apricots (dried) Cherries Fruit cocktail Grapefruit Grapes Orange Orange marmalade Peach, fresh Pear, fresh or tinned Plum Prunes Strawberries Strawberry jam	Apricots, fresh or tinned Apricot jam Banana Kiwi fruit Mango Melon Papaya Peach, canned Pineapple Raisins Sultanas	Dates, dried Lychee Watermelon
Fruit juices	Apple juice Grapefruit juice Orange juice Pineapple juice, unsweetened	Rye	

▶

	Low GI	Medium GI	High GI
Pulses	Baked beans Butter beans Chickpeas Haricot beans Kidney beans Lentils Soya beans	Broad beans	
Rice	Uncle Ben's	Basmati, boiled Brown Long grain, white	Instant Rice cakes Short grain, white Sticky
Snacks	Peanuts (contain significant fat)	Potato crisps (contain significant fat)	Popcorn
Sugars		Honey Sucrose (table sugar)	Glucose
Vegetabl es	Carrots Peas Sweet corn Sweet potato	Beetroot Small new potatoes	Parsnip Potatoes Pumpkin Swede

REFERENCES

1. Tang-Peronard, J.L., Andersen, H.R., Jensen, T.K., Heitmann, B.L., 'Endocrine-disrupting chemicals and obesity development in humans: A review', *Obesity Reviews*, 2011;12:622–36. Rezg, R., El-Fazaa, Sa., Gharbi, N., Mornagui, B., 'Bisphenol A and human chronic diseases: Current evidences, possible mechanisms, and future perspectives', *Environment International*, March 2014;64:83–90.

2. Silventoinen, K., Rokholm, B., Kaprio, J., Sorensen, T.I., 'The genetic and environmental influences on childhood obesity: A systematic review of twin and adoption studies', *International Journal of Obesity*, (London) 2010;34:29–40.

3. Llewellyn, C.H., van Jaarsveld, C.H., Plomin, R., Fisher, A., Wardle, J., 'Inherited behavioral susceptibility to adiposity in infancy: A multivariate genetic analysis of appetite and weight in the Gemini birth cohort', *American Journal of Clinical Nutrition*, 2012;95:633–9.

4. Donnelly, J.E., et al., 'A randomized, controlled, supervised, exercise trial in young overweight men and women: The Midwest Exercise Trial II (MET2)', *Contemporary Clinical Trials*, July 2012;33(4):804–10.

5. Musso, G., et al., 'Obesity, diabetes, and gut microbiota: The hygiene hypothesis expanded?', *Diabetes Care*, 2010 Oct;33(10):2277–84.

6. Hu, F., Stampfer, M., Manson, J., et al., 'Dietary fat intake and the risk of coronary heart disease in women', *New England Journal of Medicine*, 1997;337:1491–9.

7. Fujioka, K., Greenway, F., Sheard, J., Ying, Y., 'The effects of grapefruit on weight and insulin resistance: Relationship to the metabolic syndrome', *Journal of Medicinal Food*, Spring 2006;9(1):49–54.

Appendix 1

HIIT – WHAT'S THE EVIDENCE?

There is a wealth of scientific evidence for the effectiveness of HIIT in fat burning and therefore weight control. In fact, I could have filled this whole book with all the research, which incidentally is all freely available online. Below I have picked out just a few pieces of research to give you a flavour of how much scientists believe in the value of HIIT.

1. In 1994 researchers at Laval University, Quebec, found that bursts of high-intensity intermittent exercise, while burning up far fewer calories, results in nine times more fat reduction.

The abstract: http://www.ncbi.nlm.nih.gov/pubmed/8028502, Tremblay, A., Simoneau, J.A., Bouchard, C., 'Impact of exercise intensity on body fatness and skeletal muscle metabolism', *Metabolism*, 1994 Jul;43(7):814–8, Physical Activity Sciences Laboratory, Laval University, Ste-Foy, Quebec, Canada.

> The impact of two different modes of training on body fatness and skeletal muscle metabolism was investigated in young adults who were subjected to either a 20-week endurance-training (ET) program (eight men and nine women) or a 15-week high-intensity intermittent-training (HIIT) program (five men and five women). The mean estimated total energy cost of the ET program was 120.4 MJ, whereas the corresponding value for the HIIT program was

57.9 MJ. Despite its lower energy cost, the HIIT program induced a more pronounced reduction in subcutaneous adiposity compared with the ET program. When corrected for the energy cost of training, the decrease in the sum of six subcutaneous skinfolds induced by the HIIT program was ninefold greater than by the ET program. Muscle biopsies obtained in the vastus lateralis before and after training showed that both training programs increased similarly the level of the citric acid cycle enzymatic marker. On the other hand, the activity of muscle glycolytic enzymes was increased by the HIIT program, whereas a decrease was observed following the ET program. The enhancing effect of training on muscle 3-hydroxyacyl coenzyme A dehydrogenase (HADH) enzyme activity, a marker of the activity of beta-oxidation, was significantly greater after the HIIT program. In conclusion, these results reinforce the notion that for a given level of energy expenditure, vigorous exercise favors negative energy and lipid balance to a greater extent than exercise of low to moderate intensity. Moreover, the metabolic adaptations taking place in the skeletal muscle in response to the HIIT program appear to favor the process of lipid oxidation.

2. In 2006 scientists at the University of Guelph, Canada, Stirling University, Scotland, and McMaster University, Canada, showed that high-intensity aerobic interval training increases the capacity for fat oxidation during exercise in women, that is, HIIT increased the rate of body-fat burn-off. The following year another study at the same university showed that high-intensity aerobic interval training increases fat and carbohydrate metabolic capacities in human skeletal muscle, that is, HIIT increases the burning off of body fat.

The abstract: http://jap.physiology.org/content/102/4/1439, Talanian, J.L., Galloway, S.D.R., Heigenhauser, G.J.F, Bone, A. and Spriet, L.L., 'Two weeks of high-intensity aerobic interval training increases the capacity for fat oxidation during exercise in women',

Journal of Applied Physiology, 2007 Apr;102(4):1439–47, Department of Human Health and Nutritional Sciences, University of Guelph, Guelph, Ontario, Canada; Department of Sport Studies, University of Stirling, Stirling, Scotland; and Department of Medicine, McMaster University, Hamilton, Ontario, Canada.

Our aim was to examine the effects of seven high-intensity aerobic interval training (HIIT) sessions over 2 wk on skeletal muscle fuel content, mitochondrial enzyme activities, fatty acid transport proteins, peak O2 consumption (VO2 peak), and whole body metabolic, hormonal, and cardiovascular responses to exercise. Eight women (22.1 ± 0.2 yr old, 65.0 ± 2.2 kg body wt, 2.36 ± 0.24 l/min VO2 peak) performed a VO2 peak test and a 60-min cycling trial at ~60% VO2 peak before and after training. Each session consisted of ten 4-min bouts at ~90% VO2 peak with 2 min of rest between intervals. Training increased VO2 peak by 13%. After HIIT, plasma epinephrine and heart rate were lower during the final 30 min of the 60-min cycling trial at ~60% pretraining VO2 peak. Exercise whole body fat oxidation increased by 36% (from 15.0 ± 2.4 to 20.4 ± 2.5 g) after HIIT. Resting muscle glycogen and triacylglycerol contents were unaffected by HIIT, but net glycogen use was reduced during the posttraining 60-min cycling trial. HIIT significantly increased muscle mitochondrial β-hydroxyacyl-CoA dehydrogenase (15.44 ± 1.57 and 20.35 ± 1.40 mmol·min−1·kg wet mass−1 before and after training, respectively) and citrate synthase (24.45 ± 1.89 and 29.31 ± 1.64 mmol·min−1·kg wet mass−1 before and after training, respectively) maximal activities by 32% and 20%, while cytoplasmic hormone-sensitive lipase protein content was not significantly increased. Total muscle plasma membrane fatty acid-binding protein content increased significantly (25%), whereas fatty acid translocase/CD36 content was unaffected after HIIT. In summary, seven sessions of HIIT over 2 wk induced marked increases in whole body and skeletal muscle capacity for fatty acid oxidation during exercise in moderately active women.

3. In 2008 the scientists at the University of Guelph, Canada, showed that high-intensity aerobic interval training increases fat and carbohydrate metabolic capacities in human skeletal muscle, that is, HIIT increases the burning off of body fat.

The abstract: http://www.ncbi.nlm.nih.gov/pubmed/19088769, Perry, C.G., Heigenhauser, G.J., Bonen, A., Spriet, L.L., 'High-intensity aerobic interval training increases fat and carbohydrate metabolic capacities in human skeletal muscle', *Applied Physiology Nutrition and Metabolism*, 2008 Dec;33(6):1112–23. Department of Human Health and Nutritional Sciences, University of Guelph, ON N1G 2W1, Canada. perryc@uoguelph.ca.

High-intensity aerobic interval training (HIIT) is a compromise between time-consuming moderate-intensity training and sprint-interval training requiring all-out efforts. However, there are few data regarding the ability of HIIT to increase the capacities of fat and carbohydrate oxidation in skeletal muscle. Using untrained recreationally active individuals, we investigated skeletal muscle and whole-body metabolic adaptations that occurred following 6 weeks of HIIT ($\sim$1 h of 10 × 4 min intervals at $\sim$90% of peak oxygen consumption (VO2 peak), separated by 2 min rest, 3 d.week-1). A VO2 peak test, a test to exhaustion (TE) at 90% of pre-training VO2 peak, and a 1 h cycle at 60% of pre-training VO2 peak were performed pre- and post-HIIT. Muscle biopsies were sampled during the TE at rest, after 5 min, and at exhaustion. Training power output increased by 21%, and VO2 peak increased by 9% following HIIT. Muscle adaptations at rest included the following: (i) increased cytochrome c oxidase IV content (18%) and maximal activities of the mitochondrial enzymes citrate synthase (26%), beta-hydroxyacyl-CoA dehydrogenase (29%), aspartate-amino transferase (26%), and pyruvate dehydrogenase (PDH; 21%); (ii) increased FAT/CD36, FABPpm, GLUT 4, and MCT 1 and 4 transport proteins (14%-30%); and (iii) increased glycogen content (59%). Major adaptations during exercise included the following: (i) reduced glycogenolysis, lactate accumulation, and substrate phosphorylation (0–5 min of TE); (ii) unchanged PDH activation (carbohydrate oxidation; 0–5 min of TE); (iii) ~2-fold greater time during the TE; and (iv) increased fat oxidation at 60% of pre-training VO2 peak. This study demonstrated that 18 h of repeated high-intensity exercise sessions over 6 weeks (3 d.week-1) is a powerful method to increase whole-body and skeletal muscle capacities to oxidize fat and carbohydrate in previously untrained individuals.

4. Research in 2009 at Heriot-Watt University Edinburgh, Scotland, showed that HIIT substantially improves insulin action. The significance of this is that if you improve insulin action you improve fat burning.

The abstract: http://www.ncbi.nlm.nih.gov/pubmed/19175906, Babraj, J.A., Vollaard, N.B., Keast, C., Guppy, F.M., Cottrell, G., Timmons, J.A., 'Extremely short duration high intensity interval training substantially improves insulin action in young healthy males', *BMC Endocrine Disorders*, 2009 Jan 28;9:3. Translational Biomedicine, School of Engineering and Physical Sciences, Heriot-Watt University Edinburgh, Scotland, UK. j.babraj@hw.ac.uk.

BACKGROUND: Traditional high volume aerobic exercise training reduces cardiovascular and metabolic disease risk but involves a substantial time commitment. Extremely low volume high-intensity interval training (HIT) has recently been demonstrated to produce improvements to aerobic function, but it is unknown whether HIT has the capacity to improve insulin action and hence glycemic control.

METHODS: Sixteen young men (age: 21 +/- 2 y; BMI: 23.7 +/- 3.1 kg × m-2; VO2peak: 48 +/- 9 ml × kg-1 × min-1) performed 2 weeks of supervised HIT comprising of a total of 15 min of exercise (6 sessions; 4–6 × 30-s cycle sprints per session). Aerobic performance (250-kJ self-paced cycling time trial), and glucose, insulin and NEFA responses to a 75-g oral glucose load (oral glucose tolerance test; OGTT) were determined before and after training.

RESULTS: Following 2 weeks of HIT, the area under the plasma glucose, insulin and NEFA concentration-time curves were all reduced (12%, 37%, 26% respectively, all P < 0.001). Fasting plasma insulin and glucose concentrations remained unchanged, but there was a tendency for reduced fasting plasma NEFA concentrations post-training (pre: 350 +/- 36 v post: 290 +/- 39 micromol × l-1, P = 0.058). Insulin sensitivity, as measured by the Cederholm index, was improved by 23% (P < 0.01), while aerobic cycling performance improved by approximately 6% (P < 0.01).

CONCLUSION: The efficacy of a high intensity exercise protocol, involving only ~250 kcal of work each week, to substantially improve insulin action in young sedentary subjects is remarkable. This novel time-efficient training paradigm can be used as a strategy to reduce metabolic risk factors in young and middle aged sedentary populations who otherwise would not adhere to time consuming traditional aerobic exercise regimes.

5. In 2007, scientists at the University of Copenhagen, Denmark, showed that the energy expenditure associated with multiple short daily sessions, that is, HIIT, may be greater than that in a single daily session. This demonstrates that HIIT is more effective for fat burning than traditional exercise.

The abstract: http://www.ncbi.nlm.nih.gov/pubmed/17763840, Eriksen, L., Dahl-Petersen, I., Haugaard, S.B., Dela, F., 'Comparison of the effect of multiple short-duration with single long-duration exercise sessions on glucose homeostasis in type-2 diabetes mellitus', *Diabetologia.* 2007 Nov;50(11):2245–53. Epub 2007 Sep 1. Department of Biomedical Sciences, The Copenhagen Muscle Research Centre, Faculty of Health Sciences, University of Copenhagen, Blegdamsvej 3, 2200 Copenhagen, Denmark. Republished in: *Ugeskr Laeger,* 2009 Mar 9;171(11):878–80.

AIMS/HYPOTHESIS: We evaluated and compared the effects on glycaemic control of two different exercise protocols in elderly men with type 2 diabetes mellitus.

METHODS: Eighteen patients with type 2 diabetes mellitus carried out home-based bicycle training for 5 weeks. Patients were randomly assigned to one of two training programmes at 60% of maximal oxygen uptake: three 10 min sessions per day (3 × 10) or one 30 min session per day (1 × 30). Plasma insulin, C-peptide and glucose concentrations were measured during a 3 h oral glucose tolerance test (OGTT). Insulin sensitivity index (ISI(composite)), pre-hepatic insulin secretion rates (ISR) and change in insulin secretion per unit change in glucose concentrations (B(total)) were calculated.

RESULTS: Cardiorespiratory fitness increased in response to training in both groups. In group 3 × 10 (n = 9) fasting plasma glucose (p = 0.01), 120 min glucose OGTT (p = 0.04) and plasma glucose concentration areas under the curve at 120 min (p < 0.04) and 180 min (p = 0.07) decreased. These parameters remained unchanged in group 1 × 30 (n = 9). No significant changes were found in ISI(composite), ISR and B(total) in either of the exercise groups. In a matched time-control group (n = 10), glycaemic control did not change.

CONCLUSIONS/INTERPRETATION: Moderate to high-intensity training performed at 3 × 10 min/day is preferable to 1 × 30 min/day with regard to effects on glycaemic control. This is in spite of the fact that cardiorespiratory fitness increased similarly in both exercise groups. A possible explanation is that the energy expenditure associated with multiple short daily sessions may be greater than that in a single daily session.

6. Research in 2009 at McMaster University, Ontario, Canada, showed that HIIT increased capacity for glucose and fatty-acid oxidation. Increased fatty-acid oxidation results in increased fat burning.

The abstract: http://www.ncbi.nlm.nih.gov/pubmed/19112161, Gibala, M.J., McGee, S.L., Garnham, A.P., Howlett, K.F., Snow, R.J., Hargreaves, M., 'Brief intense interval exercise activates AMPK and p38 MAPK signaling and increases the expression of PGC-1alpha in human skeletal muscle', *Journal of Applied Physiology*, 2009 Mar;106(3):929–34. Epub 2008 Dec 26. Department of Kinesiology, McMaster University, Hamilton, Ontario, Canada. gibalam@mcmaster.ca.

From a cell signaling perspective, short-duration intense muscular work is typically associated with resistance training and linked to pathways that stimulate growth. However, brief repeated sessions of sprint or high-intensity interval exercise induce rapid phenotypic changes that resemble traditional endurance training. We tested the hypothesis that an acute session of intense intermittent cycle exercise would activate signaling cascades linked to mitochondrial biogenesis in human skeletal muscle. Biopsies (vastus lateralis) were obtained from six young men who performed four 30-s "all out" exercise bouts interspersed with 4 min of rest (<80 kJ total work). Phosphorylation of AMP-activated protein kinase (AMPK; subunits alpha1 and alpha2) and the p38 mitogen-activated protein kinase (MAPK) was higher ($P <$ or $= 0.05$) immediately after bout 4 vs. preexercise. Peroxisome proliferator-activated receptor-gamma coactivator-1alpha (PGC-1alpha) mRNA was increased approximately twofold above rest after 3 h of recovery (P <or= 0.05); however, PGC-1alpha protein content was unchanged. In contrast, phosphorylation of protein kinase B/Akt (Thr(308) and Ser(473)) tended to decrease, and downstream targets linked to hypertrophy (p70 ribosomal S6 kinase and 4E binding protein 1) were unchanged after exercise and recovery. We conclude that signaling through AMPK and p38 MAPK to PGC-1alpha may explain in part the metabolic remodeling induced by low-volume intense interval exercise, including mitochondrial biogenesis and an increased capacity for glucose and fatty acid oxidation.

GRAPEFRUIT INTERACTIONS

Grapefruit can interact with some prescription medications, either to increase the effect of those medications or to produce side effects. Something in grapefruit, perhaps a bioflavonoid, inhibits an enzyme called CYP 3A4, in the wall of the intestine, and this enzyme is important for the breakdown of hundreds of medications. When the effectiveness of CYP 3A4 is compromised, blood levels of these drugs can rise and cause undesirable side effects. This happens only with drugs taken by mouth – not those given by injection or via a skin patch – and the effect may last for as long as two days. If you are on any of the following drugs you should discuss with your doctor whether it is safe to eat grapefruit. He or she will help you to monitor any possible interactions if it is decided you can eat the fruit.

Drugs that may interact with grapefruit in some people are:

▶ Some calcium channel blockers, such as felodipine (Plendil), nicardipine (Cardene), nifedipine (Adalat), verapamil

▶ Some heart drugs, such as amiodarone (Cordarone), quinidine

▶ Some statins, such as atorvastatin (Lipitor), simvastatin (Zocor) but not pravastatin (Pravachol) and fluvastatin (Lescol).

▶ The blood-pressure drug, losartan (Cozaar)

▶ Some sleeping pills and anti-anxiety drugs, such as buspirone, (Buspar), diazepam (Valium), triazolam (Halcion)

▶ Some transplant drugs, such as cyclosporine, tacrolimus and sirolimus

▶ Some antidepressants, such as nefazodone (Serzone) and trazodone (Desyrel)

▶ The antipsychotic, clomipramine (Anafranil)

▶ The cortosone-like drug, methylprednisolone

▶ The impotence (erectile dysfunction) drug, sildenafil (Viagra)

▶ The asthma drug, montelukast (Singulair)

▶ The Alzheimer's drug, donepezil (Aricept)

▶ The breast cancer drug, tamoxifen (Nolvadex)

▶ The prostate drug, tamsulosin (Flomax)

▶ The antihistamines, loratadine (Claritin) and fexofenadine (Allegra)

▶ Some oestrogens

▶ Some birth-control pills

▶ The HIV/AIDS drugs, ritonavir (Norvir), saquinavir (Fortovase, Invirase)

▶ The epilepsy drug, carbamazepine (Tegretol)

INDEX